ALSO BY ERIC LAX

On Being Funny

Woody Allen, A Biography

Life and Death on 10 West

Bogart (with A. M. Sperber)

THE MOLD IN DR. FLOREY'S COAT

THE MOLD IN
DR. FLOREY'S COAT

THE STORY OF THE PENICILLIN MIRACLE

ERIC LAX

A JOHN MACRAE BOOK
HENRY HOLT AND COMPANY | NEW YORK

Henry Holt and Company, LLC
Publishers since 1866
115 West 18th Street
New York, New York 10011

Henry Holt® is a registered trademark of
Henry Holt and Company, LLC.

Library of Congress Cataloging-in-Publication Data
Lax, Eric.
　　The mold in Dr. Florey's coat : the story of the penicillin miracle /
Eric Lax.
　　　　p.　cm.
Includes bibliographical references and index.
　　ISBN 0-8050-6790-6
　　1. Penicillin—History—Popular works.　I., Title: Mold in Doctor Florey's coat.
II. Title.
　　RM666.P35L39 2004
　　615'.3295654—dc22　　　　　　　　　　　　　　　　　　　　2003056685

First Edition 2004

Designed by Kelly S. Too

Printed in the United States of America
3　5　7　9　10　8　6　4

For my son John

"The more intelligent the question you ask of Mother Nature, the more intelligent will be her reply."

—SIR CHARLES SHERRINGTON

CONTENTS

INTRODUCTION:
THE RECLAIMED LIFE

On March 14, 1942, thirty-one-year-old Anne Miller lay in New Haven Hospital dying of blood poisoning. She had developed a bacterial infection following a miscarriage a month before, a then common complication that quickly could turn fatal. For all those weeks her temperature swung between 103 and 106 degrees F (39.4 and 41.1 degrees C), often leaving her delirious as her condition worsened and her body wasted away from her inability to eat. Blood transfusions, surgery, and many doses of the recently developed sulfa drugs all failed to kill the streptococcus that had colonized her blood.

Her doctor, John Bumstead of the Yale clinical faculty, was about out of hope for her when he remembered a passing conversation with Dr. John Fulton, another of his patients, who was lying ill in a nearby room. Fulton and his wife were friends of Howard Florey, an Oxford University scientist who headed the group that was developing an almost unknown substance called penicillin, which was many times more powerful against bacteria than any known drug. The devastation and the crippling of industry caused by World War II made further production and testing in England difficult, so in 1941 Florey and his colleague Norman Heatley had come to the United States to try to persuade American drug companies to work on this potentially miraculous but still unproven medicine. Heatley had even stayed on to help the New Jersey pharmaceutical company Merck manufacture penicillin.

Bumstead beseeched Fulton to help him get some of the drug for Mrs. Miller. Fulton, a champion of Florey's research, knew the chairman of the Committee on Chemotherapy in Washington, D.C., which controlled all important medicines during World War II; after Fulton's call he authorized Merck to release 5.5 g of penicillin—about a teaspoonful. It was half of the entire amount in the United States.

The tiny cache of raw antibiotic was soon delivered to Mrs. Miller's room, where it was passed through an extrafine filter to remove impurities and dissolved in a saline solution. No one was certain of the appropriate dose, so a small one was injected by an intern, at three P.M.

Her doctors waited for a possible negative reaction, but when after four hours there was none, a larger dose was administered. When the second dose also caused no harmful reaction, all other medication was discontinued and penicillin was injected every four hours. By midnight her temperature was down to 100 degrees. By nine A.M. the next day, it was normal for the first time in a month. She began to eat hearty meals, again for the first time in weeks. Within twenty-four hours, the deadly bacterial growth in her blood had disappeared. After a month-long convalescence, during which Mrs. Miller received more penicillin manufactured by Merck, she went home and lived a pleasant life until she died in 1999, at age ninety.

Four patients in Oxford had been cured by penicillin several months earlier, but Anne Miller was arguably the first patient pulled back from death's door by the drug. Her reclaimed life marks a revolution in medicine that has touched virtually everyone on Earth.

In the fifth century B.C., Herodotus noted in his *History* that every Babylonian was an amateur physician, because the sick were laid out in the street so that any passerby might offer advice for a cure. For the next twenty-four hundred years that was as good an approach to infection as any, since all doctors' remedies against it were almost uniformly powerless. Until the middle of the twentieth century, mothers routinely died from infections following childbirth; children were killed by diarrhea, scarlet fever, measles, and tonsillitis; and anyone who survived other onslaughts often was taken by pneumonia or meningitis. Soldiers most commonly died not from war injuries but from resulting infections such as septicemia and gangrene. Away from the battlefield, boils, abscesses, and carbuncles were common portals for life-threatening illness; the smallest cut could lead to a fatal infection. For much of human history, sex brought painful aftereffects in gonorrhea and eventually death in syphilis. There were a few antidotes to infection: vaccination against smallpox with cowpox vaccine, first done in 1796; the introduction of antiseptics in 1865; and the advent of sulfa drugs in 1935. Yet arrayed against these were the menacing presences of scarlet fever, typhoid fever, rheumatic fever, tuberculosis, cholera, plague, typhus, dysentery, and a catalogue of other diseases for which the doctor's best treatment was a soothing bedside manner and a steady dose of optimism; skillfully administered, this lasted the patients until they died.

All this changed in 1940, when Howard Florey, Ernst Chain, Norman Heatley, and fewer than a half-dozen others at Oxford produced penicillin. They performed their work on a minuscule budget with makeshift equipment during the most perilous time for England in World War II. The imminent possibility that the Nazis would invade the country meant that the scientists might have to destroy their work on a few hours' notice to keep it from enemy hands, and they hatched a brilliantly simple plan in the event that happened. With the hope that at least one of the team would be able to find refuge and continue the work on *Penicillium notatum,* the particular mold that spawned penicillin, Florey and four of his colleagues rubbed some of its spores in their clothes. Spores are hearty stuff, and, if necessary, those *Penicillium* spores could lie undetected and dormant for years and then be revived for further study. The invasion, of course, never occurred. Within two years they had something other than optimism for doctors to administer to their patients.

The development of penicillin was the culmination of advances large and small that began in biblical times. Just what caused infection was so unclear for millennia that a common explanation was simply to attribute epidemics to the wrath of the gods. Hippocrates, the Greek physician born in 460 B.C. and famous for the oath taken by new doctors to first do no harm, made a step toward understanding in his book *Airs, Waters and Places,* which detailed his observations of the relation between physical influences and illness. The Book of Leviticus (14:33–53) specifically details how to segregate lepers to avoid contact with them; careful observers had noticed that diseases could be passed from one person to another not only through physical contact but also by items used in common, such as utensils and clothing.

The first person to see and identify a microbe was Antoni van Leeuwenhoek, a Dutch draper and lens grinder. In 1675, he invented the microscope, a magnifying glass attached to a three-inch-long piece of brass. Even with so primitive an instrument, Leeuwenhoek saw moving objects in a drop of his own saliva, which left him reeling from the notion that these things were in his body. Because the objects moved, he presumed they were alive, and he wrote of them as "little animals, a thousand times smaller than the eye of a full-grown louse."

The development of the compound microscope in the 1830s enabled scientists to see that large numbers of single-cell, rod-shaped organisms are present in our bodies and most everywhere else. Their shape led to their being named *bacteria,* which is derived from the Greek for *stick* or *staff,* in the 1840s.

Meanwhile, Edward Jenner demonstrated in rural England in 1796 that people inoculated with cowpox were immune to smallpox. Thus, an illness that killed millions was curtailed, although neither the nature of infection nor how vaccination worked was then understood.

The English surgeon Joseph Lister's introduction in 1865 of "antiseptic" in operating rooms vastly lowered the almost 50 percent fatality rate of patients whose surgery was successful but who died from subsequent infection.

Louis Pasteur's discovery in 1877 that killer organisms rendered harmless prevented infection by active bacteria showed that immunity against any number of infectious diseases was possible. Still, death remained a common result of bacterial invasions, which could colonize the blood or fulminate in even the smallest wound.

In 1880, the German bacteriologist Robert Koch discovered that microorganisms were the root of disease, not the result. By the end of the nineteenth century, microorganisms responsible for many diseases in humans and animals had been identified, and it was clear that bacteria played a major role in human life, and death.

Then in the fall of 1928, Dr. Alexander Fleming discovered penicillin's potential against bacteria in a chance observation while examining a stray mold that had bloomed in a culture dish of the bacteria *Staphylococcus* in his London laboratory. *Staphylococcus,* like its cousin *Streptococcus*, can do great damage. When people speak of a "staph infection" or "strep throat," they are referring to these microbes, which are as small as a quarter of a millionth of an inch in diameter. In part they are classified according to how they divide when multiplying in colonies. When they divide regularly, they form a chain: streptococci. When they divide irregularly, they bunch like grapes: staphylococci. There are about 150 species of these two groups, and each group causes its own mayhem. *Staphylococcus* is found in abscesses and blood poisoning; *Streptococcus* spreads inflammation.

The usefulness of Jenner's, Lister's, and Pasteur's discoveries were almost immediately clear, but the importance of the mold that led to the first antibiotic was not. Fleming found that the antibacterial substance the penicillin mold produced was elusive by nature and seemingly impossible to isolate from the mixture he cultivated it in. During the process of separating the drug from the broth it grows in, its magical properties vanished; penicillin was the Scarlet Pimpernel of medical research. Fleming had made a vital find, but he made little progress beyond that and eventually abandoned his work on it. He is rather like a man who, say, discovered sparkling stuff in the water at Sutter's Mill in California in 1848, saw that it looked like gold, but was unable to mine it. A dozen years passed before the Florey-led group of Oxford scientists was able to advance beyond Fleming's observation.

None of the scientists involved with penicillin set out to change human history, but indeed they did. In retrospect, how their remarkable breakthrough was accomplished makes it all the more extraordinary, and how credit for it was given—or misplaced—all the more interesting.

There are four people at the heart of the penicillin story: Fleming,

Florey, Heatley, and Ernst Chain, a key member of the Oxford team. They worked before most of us were alive, in a manner and time far different from our own. It was an era when physicians had few weapons to fight disease; when experiments were carried out with crude, often homemade instruments; when financial gain was not a driving force of science; and when a scratch from a rose thorn could start a downward spiral to death.

1

THE QUIET SCOT

Anyone able to associate a name with the development of penicillin almost invariably thinks of Alexander Fleming, whose fame in the middle of the twentieth century was such that he was a celebrity on every continent of Earth and on the Moon as well, where a crater was named for him. Those who don't recall Fleming often but incorrectly think credit lies with Louis Pasteur, Marie Curie, or Jonas Salk. But Howard Florey, Ernst Chain, and Norman Heatley, who turned quirky mold into the life-saving drug, are virtually unknown.

However, penicillin's development does begin with Fleming, a keen observer, a dexterous, even playful, manipulator of microorganisms and scientific equipment, and a member of the Inoculation Department at St. Mary's Hospital in London, just up Praed Street from Paddington Station.

The seventh of eight children, Fleming was born August 6, 1881, near Darvel, Ayrshire, in southwestern Scotland. His father, Hugh, kept several hundred sheep on the family's eight-hundred-acre farm in the almost barren hills and valleys, where Alec led an active outdoor life that honed his natural skill of observation. He had light hair and a flattened nose, and he grew to be slightly less than five-foot-six. His most noticeable features were large, strikingly blue eyes. They were also his most disconcerting, in that they often seemed focused through rather than on the person with whom he was talking. This unease he created in others was compounded by his lack of conversational skills.

Later in life, he had friends across a wide expanse of society, but for the most part, one noted, "He was not a conversationalist and awkward silences were sometimes broken by awkward remarks . . . talking with him was like playing tennis with a man who, whenever you knocked the ball over to his side, put it in his pocket." More reticent than rude or shy, he made few close friends other than his four brothers; he was particularly devoted to Robert, two years his junior.

Hugh died in 1888, leaving his oldest son tenancy of the farm and most of his other children without prospects. One by one, they moved to London. Alec left school the summer he turned fourteen and joined the exodus south to live with his brother Thomas, a doctor thirteen years his senior who specialized in ophthalmology, and their sister Mary and brother John. Robert soon followed, and the two youngsters enrolled at the Regent Street Polytechnic Institute, founded by the philanthropist Quentin Hogg in 1892 "for the promotion of industrial skill, general knowledge, health and well being of young men belonging to the poorer classes."

Because it had been difficult for Thomas to establish his practice, he recommended that Alec might have an easier life if he took commercial courses for what Thomas thought would be a safer career in business. Alec found the studies easy; he moved up four classes in his first two weeks and at sixteen had passed all his courses. He landed a job as a junior clerk with the America Line, one of the leading fleets in the Atlantic trade, doing the mind- and finger-numbing work of copying letters and documents, filling in ledgers, and preparing cargo manifests.

Alec refreshed himself by joining in family competitions arranged by Thomas. Everyone anted a penny for winner-take-all contests in almost anything that could be contested: history, math, and geography; poker, bridge, and snooker; bowling, croquet, and even the occasional intrafamily boxing match.

He was a good shot as well. So many British soldiers were sent to South Africa to fight the Boer War from 1899 to 1902 that volunteers were sought to man home regiments based on county or regional affiliation. In 1900, Alec, a natural athlete and a good shot, and Robert enlisted in the London Scottish Rifle Volunteers, a brigade that was as much a club as it was a fighting force; Alec joined their rifle and water polo teams.

That same year, the Fleming children's uncle died, leaving them each the considerable sum of £250. Thomas invested his share in a better office. His practice soon flourished, and he encouraged Alec to use his promised inheritance (he could not receive it until he was twenty-one) to attend medical school. Alec, now nearly twenty, more anxious to escape a dead-end job than he was enamored of medicine, agreed. That he was two or three years older than the others beginning their medical studies and singularly unqualified by his previous education did not strike him as drawbacks. He discovered that a diploma from the London College of Preceptors was regarded as the equal of more formal schooling, and he hired a tutor for evening studies. In July 1901, he took the medical school entrance exams in seventeen subjects that included three kinds of math, Latin, French, English, geology, physiology, scripture, and shorthand. He scored at or near the top in every one.

Entitled to enter any of the twelve London medical schools, Alec chose St. Mary's, for reasons apparently no more complicated than it was the one nearest home and because he and others of the Scottish Rifle team had once played water polo against the team from the hospital's medical school. He promptly won the entrance scholarship exam; the £145 prize paid for his tuition and equipment. It was the first of more than a dozen prizes he would win in examinations that comprised every field of medical study. Despite his reticence, he became a member of the Debating Society and of the Dramatic Society. His relatively short height often relegated him to women's parts; the two feminine leads in one production were Fleming and Charles McMoran Wilson, who in 1920 became dean of the St. Mary's Hospital Medical School and, in 1943, became Lord Moran, Winston Churchill's personal physician. This association would play a pivotal role when it came time to apportion credit for the development of penicillin.

At the turn of the twentieth century, surgeons were at the top of the medical profession, and, in January 1905, Fleming passed the examination to become a fellow of the Royal College of Surgeons. His

interest was logical, considering his dexterous hands and great knowledge of anatomy—he won the Anatomy Prize in 1902 as well as the
Senior Anatomy Prize in 1904—but, despite his ability and qualification, he never performed an operation, preferring research instead.

After Fleming completed his studies in 1906, he joined the Inoculation Department to bide his time while he settled on a specialty. He
stayed forty-nine years.

The Inoculation Department was a fiefdom with no equal in British
medicine. The department was independent of both the hospital and
the medical school and earned its own income from the treatment of
private patients and the sale of vaccines it prepared and sold to doctors
through the pharmaceutical firm Parke, Davis and Company. A notice
on the label assured doctor and patient that the product was prepared
"under the supervision of the Director, Sir Almroth Wright, MD FRS,
etc." The department also relied on the generosity of its patrons,
among them Arthur Balfour, the prime minister from 1902 to 1905.
It paid rent to the hospital for its space and in return was given a
wing of the hospital for laboratories and a ward of patients to treat.
In effect, it was the first private clinical research institute in England.

Almroth Wright, the multidegreed director of the Inoculation
Department, was a large, imposing man with hard eyes, a walrus mustache, and equally imposing views. Wright was one of the foremost
medical men of his time—in the 1890s, he developed the vaccine for
typhoid—and one of the most controversial. His admirers revered him,
his detractors called him "Sir Almost Wright" or "Sir Always Wrong,"
and he reveled in any attention, whether positive or negative. Wright
was outspoken in the extreme in his disdain of medicine-as-usual, an
opinion shared by George Bernard Shaw, who exaggerated Wright in
the character of Sir Colenso Ridgeon, the physician in his 1906 satire
The Doctor's Dilemma, who must choose between saving the life of
"an honest decent man, but is he any use?" and "a rotten blackguard,
but he's a genuine source of pretty and pleasant and good things."

In 1909, Fleming devised a method of testing for syphilis using only
a drop or two of blood rather than the larger amount required for the
eponymous test invented three years earlier by the German pathologist
August von Wassermann. The three papers on the method that Flem-

ing published in the next year brought him patients—very welcome because of his meager salary—and requests from other doctors for consultation. Then, in 1910, the German researcher Paul Ehrlich developed "606" (the first 605 compounds he tested were useless) for the treatment of syphilis. Though later called Salvarsan by physicians, it was more popularly known as the "Magic Bullet." It was the first chemically synthesized chemotherapeutic agent, which is to say, it fights a disease in every part of the body and not just where it is applied, as is the case with an antiseptic liquid or ointment.

The practice of medicine at the beginning of the twentieth century often included treatment of the diseases associated with syphilis over its decades-long course. Salvarsan offered the possibility of curing millions. Ehrlich, a friend of Wright's, sent him some of the first samples of the drug for trials on English patients. Wright had little faith that chemicals would prove the best treatments for disease, so he passed on the "606" to Fleming and Leonard Colebrook, another member of the department. By 1911, Fleming had begun giving shots of "606" to some of his private patients.

Administering the drug was a cumbersome and dangerous process. Treatment generally lasted for a year, and Salvarsan, a compound of arsenic, was so nearly toxic that it could be given only once a week. Syringes of the day were made of thick glass; their metal plungers fit so badly that often whatever was injected spewed out of the top as well as through the broad needle. The powdered drug had to be mixed in at least 600 cc's of water—about twenty ounces. If this massive amount was not injected into the arm properly, the drug escaped into the surrounding tissue. If enough did, the drug would kill the tissue and the arm might have to be amputated to prevent further damage or even death. Fleming's surgical training made him adept at handling the cumbersome hypodermic equipment, and it was soon well known that his dexterity reduced the unpleasant and dangerous side effects that resulted from less skillful injections. His private practice became lucrative.

Apart from his skill as a clinician, Fleming the researcher had a curious and frolicsome mind. "I play with microbes," he once said. "There are, of course, many rules to this play . . . but when you have acquired knowledge and experience it is very pleasant to break the rules and to be able to find something nobody had thought of."

Fleming well knew that different bacteria take on different hues as they grow, and he was adept at carefully planting various microbes on a plate of agar—the waxy, gelatinous laboratory food trough for bacteria—so that when they bloomed, the plate turned into a colorful painting of, say, a ballerina in a red skirt or a mother nursing her baby with a bottle. Arranging such scenes required a deep understanding of the peculiarities of bacterial growth and coloration, as well as the imagination to see a finished picture as he planted the microbes: the drawings developed like a slow-motion Polaroid photo, with the color appearing only after the bacteria began to divide.

Some of Fleming's contemporaries felt this whimsy lacked the dignity and seriousness appropriate to the high-minded work of science, but many important discoveries had an underpinning of play. Albert Michelson, the first American to win a Nobel Prize in physics, measured the speed of light in 1878 with $10 worth of apparatus. He said he liked to experiment "because it is so much fun!" When a visitor to the lab of the Danish physicist Niels Bohr told him with some disgust, "In your institute nobody takes anything seriously," Bohr answered, "That's quite true, and even applies to what you just said."

Bacteria are everywhere. A human body is host to between five hundred and a thousand species, with more than two hundred of these in the mouth alone. There are 10 trillion cells in a human body and more than ten times that number of bacterial cells in the digestive tract; there are more bacteria in one person's gut than there have been humans on Earth.

Only about one in one thousand species of these microbes is harmful to humans. The rest are productive citizens of our corporate bodies and together constitute a support and maintenance group. We would not be human without bacteria. Some aid in digestion and development, others eat carbohydrates that the body can't digest; some initiate the growth of the network of capillaries that move blood, and still others ensure that blood flows properly to the intestine.

But as in any society, sometimes the good turn bad. Mobile bits of DNA can wander on their chromosomes, picking up new genes from other organisms and morph benign bacteria into drug-resistant troublemakers. From the bacterial point of view, of course, human bodies are simply their homes and places of business, and these changes allow them to stay well and prosper.

Bacterial life is a simple combination of survival and reproduction, achieved through constant warfare with other microbes for space and food. Bacteria in the soil are particularly beneficial to farming, just as the bacteria in our bodies provide a multitude of housekeeping services. Bacteria that live in humans and other animals but don't cause disease are called commensals. Those that cause disease are called pathogens. Until the advent of antibiotics, pathogens were unstoppable serial killers.

Fleming's inventive approach to his work proved valuable in the struggle against pathogens. During World War I, Sir Alfred Keough, the director general of the Army Medical Services, wanted better control of wound infection. Wright accepted his request to study how best to accomplish this, and, along with Fleming and several others of his St. Mary's staff, he was given an army commission and sent to France. In October 1914, Lieutenant Fleming was billeted in the casino at Boulogne, a recreation center turned British Army General Hospital on the north coast, under the command of Colonel Wright. The main floors of the building, parceled into high-ceilinged, ornate, and once elegant rooms, were now wards filled with soldiers crazed from high fevers brought on by infection. Many of the wounded had spent a day or more lying on the field of battle because so vast a number were injured—in 1914, an average of twelve hundred patients a day was handled by the staff of clearing stations designed to help two hundred. Then once in Boulogne, they sometimes had to wait days for surgery.

The accepted treatment of open wounds was not to clean and suture them but instead to pack them with cloth bandages usually soaked in carbolic acid, the foul-smelling antiseptic widely used to clean sewers that Lister found was lethal to microbes at a strength just tolerable to human tissue. The bandages hastily applied by medics in the field were more factories of infection than aids to healing. As the bandages became sodden with pus, they were replaced with new ones. This treatment made sense, at least in theory; Lister's use of chemicals destroyed bacteria on the surface of skin and on operating utensils and also was effective in preventing infection, so it was logical to think it would also cure established infection. It didn't. Yet even after the rampant infection of soldiers' wounds in France showed that in many cases antiseptics were almost useless, Sir William Watson Cheyne, the president of the Royal College of Surgeons, stubbornly advocated the use of stronger and stronger chemical antiseptics because they had been effective during the Boer War.

Soldiers continued to die in droves from infection because the weapons and the terrain of this war were markedly different. The fighting in South Africa took place on rocky, sandy ground unaltered and unadulterated by cultivation and fertilizers and therefore not particularly prone to cause infection; the battlefields in France were muddy stews of earth and horse manure, and the trenches where the soldiers sheltered were cesspools that were spawning grounds for deadly bacteria. The guns of the Boer War shot high-speed bullets that left a clean wound. Nothing about World War I was clean. Uniforms soaked up the bacteria. Shrapnel from explosive shells drove pieces of uniform into a wound and embedded bacteria in tissues or bone so far beyond the wound itself that antiseptics were not strong enough to reach them. The most efficient killers of all were bacteria that were invisible to the naked eye and often had only to rely on the power of weapons or even the soldiers themselves for their transport.

Of the 10 million soldiers killed in World War I, about half died not from bombs or shrapnel or bullets or gas but rather from infection in an often relatively minor wound. The fertilizer on the farm fields that became battlefields promoted the growth of such common soil bacteria as *Streptococcus* and *Staphylococcus,* which produce pus and infection in humans. Other, deadlier bacteria thrived as well, among them those that cause tetanus, a usually fatal locking of the muscles, and septicemia, or blood poisoning. Worse was the bacterium *Clostridium welchii (perfringens),* a cause of gangrene, which begins in the dead tissue of a wound but quickly spreads to healthy muscles and bloats a wide area; within a few hours an entire limb can become grotesquely inflated, the dead flesh greenish-black and putrid.

The expanding gas brings on excruciating pain, sweating, fever, and quick death. Scores of thousands of soldiers had an arm or leg amputated in an effort to stop the spread of gangrene, but in many cases it was too late to save their lives; the bacteria had already coursed ahead of the surgeon's saw and poisoned the blood. Infected soldiers were alert to the time of death. As Keough put it in 1914, "We have, in this war, gone straight back to all the septic infections of the Middle Ages."

Fleming, then thirty-three, spent his time in the attic of the casino where the local fencing team had practiced and which was now a jury-rigged lab largely the result of his ingenuity. A master of improvisation, he used gas cans and pumps to bring in water; made incubators from paraffin stoves; used a foot bellows to power a glass-blowing burner for shaping lab equipment; and tweaked Bunsen burners so that they could be powered by alcohol. He later said that the lab at Boulogne was one of the best he ever worked in; he abhorred overly equipped labs: "I have known research workers reduced to impotence by apparatus so fine and elaborate that they spend all their time playing with it. . . . If the palace wins, he is lost."

In his lab, Fleming examined wound swabs, bullets, shell fragments, and shreds of uniform, as well as dead tissue and bits of bone removed by surgeons. Fleming's examination of fabric from soldiers' uniforms uncontaminated by blood or pus showed that among this presumably clean material 15 percent carried staphylococci, 30 percent bore tetanus bacilli, 40 percent had streptococci—and that 90 percent of the samples grew *Clostridium welchii,* which caused gangrene.

Fleming realized that even though many of the germs were being killed, many others lay protected in ragged tears of the wound, and that the dressings were no more than what Wright called "a putrefactive poultice." In a simple but elegant demonstration Fleming took an ordinary glass test tube, heated it in order to pull out spiked pieces so that the end of the tube resembled a hollow medieval mace (the jagged edges simulated a shrapnel wound), then filled it with fecal bacteria-laced liquid to approximate what would enter in a battle injury and incubated it at body temperature overnight. The next day the now vile-smelling liquid, thick and opaque with massive bacterial growth, was discarded. Fleming then refilled the tube with an antiseptic solution and incubated it for a day. After that, he replaced the antiseptic with a culture medium that would allow any remaining bacteria to grow. As he predicted, within hours the bacteria were back in full force. Antiseptics may have worked perfectly on the flat surface of a glass test tube or in a clear-cut bullet hole, but they were abysmal in the mess of a shrapnel wound, where bacteria hid in the deep crevasses of the ripped flesh, and blood and pus carried the medicine away. Of course, there was a vast difference between preventing infection and overcoming it once it was established; it was to the latter that Fleming would devote his career.

The conventional story of how Fleming discovered penicillin is heart-warmingly simple and serendipitous, which perhaps is why it has persisted for so long, even though it is impossible: Fleming, an expert on *Staphylococcus,* was asked to contribute to a section on the microbe for the second of a nine-volume work, *A System of Bacteriology,* to be published by the government-funded Medical Research Council (MRC). *Staphylococcus aureus,* which usually is a golden yellow when it is cultured in the lab, is one of the most troublesome strains to humans. There was some evidence that mutant strains identifiable by their different colors were produced if, after only twenty-four hours of incubation, the bacteria were then allowed to grow at room temperature.

This interested Fleming, and not just because it might give him additional colors to use in his bacteria paintings. Beginning in 1927, he and his research assistant, D. Merlin Pryce, worked in his ten-foot-by-twelve-foot lab that filled a turreted corner on the second floor of St. Mary's, experimenting with colonies of the bacteria that they grew in covered petri dishes. From time to time they would have to remove the top of the dish to better observe the microbes.

All straightforward so far. What happened next is less so.

In February 1928, Pryce moved on to other work, and for the next five months Fleming continued on alone. It was warm that summer, and sometimes he would open one of the small windows for relief from the heat. At the end of July, shortly before his forty-seventh birthday, Fleming left with his wife, Sarah, known as Sareen, and their four-year-old son, Robert, for a month's vacation at The Dhoon, their comfortable country house in Suffolk not far from the Newmarket racecourse. Because lab space was at a premium, a colleague used Fleming's room while he was away.

Before he left, Fleming piled two or three dozen of his seeded culture plates at the end of the workbench, out of the sunlight and away from the work area. Sometime after he returned in late August or early September, he looked at what he'd left behind. He uncovered the petri dishes one by one, made notes of anything interesting, then placed the dishes in a shallow tray of disinfectant to kill the bacteria and make the dishes safe for cleaning. There were so many dishes, however, that a large number of them were stacked above the fluid.

As Fleming was doing this, Pryce stopped by to say hello and to see what progress had been made. Fleming randomly chose a few of the dishes in the tray that were above the disinfectant and showed them to Pryce. As he was about to hand Pryce one of the plates, something caught his eye.

"That's funny," he said.

A blue-green moon of mold shone over a sea of tiny islets of staphylococci. Nothing funny there; molds were and are the bane of bacteriologists. Because the dishes had to be opened so often, they were prey to contamination by spores floating in the air.

Mold and bacteria may seem closely related—they both decompose dead organic material—but they belong to two different biological groups. Bacteria and blue-green algae belong to a diverse group of primitive organisms called prokaryotes; protozoa, plants, animals, and fungi, which produce mold, are part of a more developed group called eukaryotes.

Looking more closely, Fleming now noticed that no bacteria surrounded the mold. That *was* odd, and for some distance away from the mold, there were only dead transparent cells. It was like Joshua at Jericho. Something in the mold had made the cell walls tumble down and thus caused the microbes to die. That something would eventually lead to antibiotics.

So what's wrong with this story? There is no question that Fleming observed the penicillin effect. The problem is, it is impossible to discover penicillin in the way he himself described it.

Penicillin doesn't actually kill bacteria in the way that a bullet in the heart kills a human being. Rather, it causes the cell walls to disintegrate during mitosis—division—and disables bacteria's ability to replicate. The bacteria die as a result.

The sparse details Fleming later wrote of his discovery don't help much: "On a plate planted with staphylococci a colony of mould appeared. After about two weeks it was seen that the colonies of staphylococci near the mould colony were degenerate." But if the bacteria had been planted first and taken root, penicillin could not have grown. The bacteria would have inhibited it, rather than the other way around. In a petri dish, penicillin—a fungus—must be established before colonies of bacteria in order to work its wonder.

There are two additional problems. One involves timing. Fleming supposedly took a five-week vacation that summer, but according to his own paper on penicillin, the mold appeared after two weeks. How would he have known? Moreover, in the final three weeks of Fleming's holiday, the mold would have overgrown the petri dish, not just established some colonies.

The second problem involves Fleming's notebooks. It was not until October 30—nearly two months after Fleming's return to St. Mary's—that he makes any mention in his lab book about penicillin, and that is of a completed experiment, not an accidental find. There are no known records of the date Fleming returned from his vacation, no pertinent notes in his lab book, no letters or diaries that cast light on what really happened between the time he returned and the notations of the completed experiment at the end of October. Moreover, the conventional account of how Fleming discovered penicillin—his return from vacation, Pryce's visit, the observation of antibacterial action in a discarded petri dish—was not published until 1944, after Florey and his colleagues had proven the dramatic power of penicillin and the drug was of intense public interest. The account is a convenient one. But after sixteen years, memories are often flawed.

The question of how a spore of penicillin mold managed to grow on a dish of staphylococcus was best answered by Dr. Ronald Hare in 1968, and described in his book *The Birth of Penicillin*. Hare entered

St. Mary's Medical School in 1919 and then worked as a researcher in the Inoculation Department for many years.

Hare dismisses the notion that the mold spore came through an open window in Fleming's lab for the simple reason that "the window was seldom if ever opened . . . the room would have been too noisy. Praed Street is a narrow canyon that so magnifies the roar of traffic in any room facing on it that ordinary speech becomes almost inaudible." Nor, he adds, would a good bacteriologist work near an open window because windows are the easiest routes for contaminants to enter the room. Fleming's lab has been preserved as a museum and looks today as it did seventy-five years ago. It takes only a moment to see how difficult it would have been for someone of Fleming's short height to lean across the lab bench that runs across three walls and open a window even if he wanted to.

A far more likely route for the mold spore was up the stairwell from the workroom of the Irish scientist C. J. La Touche, on the floor below Fleming. La Touche worked with molds—the name of his specialty is mycology—and a stray spore could easily have wafted up and through the usually open door to Fleming's lab. In fact, La Touche had in his collection a mold that matched the one Fleming found.

Repeated attempts by Fleming and others to replicate the growth of penicillin under the conditions he described failed. Hare deduced a reason why. In 1968, he gathered the weather records for July, August, and September 1928. From July 28 to August 7, the temperature in London rose above 68 degrees Fahrenheit only twice, and then not by much. Mold grows at room temperature; bacteria grow at body temperature. If Fleming had not incubated the dish seeded with staphylococci, it would have remained dormant, and the mold would have had a chance to establish itself before the weather turned warmer, only then allowing the bacteria to grow.

While this offers a plausible way for penicillin to grow and attack bacteria, tying it only to Fleming's vacation requires multiple coincidences: a stray mold spore; an unincubated plate of bacteria; a drop in temperature at precisely the right time to inhibit the bacteria's growth; Fleming's return from vacation in time to see the mold's effectiveness before it overran the plate; and his luck in reexamining a petri dish he has put on the stack of dishes to be cleaned in the tub of disinfectant. Then there is the question of why two months passed before Fleming wrote anything about penicillin in his notebook. Additionally, Fleming's later paper on penicillin is opaque on a variety of important points. It is impossible to tell from it what species of staphylococcus he was studying; how long the plate had been on his workbench; what type of medium it was growing in; and whether he had incubated the plate.

No amount of reconstruction will give a definite answer, but the physiologist, science historian, and MacArthur fellow Robert Scott Root-Bernstein in his book *Discovering* methodically establishes the most plausible explanation, which is that Fleming's attention was on lysozyme, a substance of lesser antibiotic power that he had discovered seven years earlier.

Unlike the discovery of penicillin, the details of Fleming's discovery of lysozyme are unambiguous. In the midst of a head cold in November 1921, Fleming put some of the mucus from his runny nose on a plate of agar and added it to the clutter of culture dishes on his workbench. Later, when he saw what had grown on it, he said to his colleague V. D. Allison, "This is interesting." (Fleming's laconic exclamations at his eureka moments reflected his understated personality.)

Along with the usual mixture of organisms Fleming noticed that there were also colonies of bacteria that were dissolving. He isolated some of them and after substantial work found this dissolving agent not only in nasal secretions but also in egg whites, turnips, bronchial mucus, human tears, and a significant number of plant and animal tissues; pike's eggs turned out to be a particularly rich source.

Beyond his own searches—Fleming found evidence that the lysozyme in a dog's saliva is stronger than that in a human's—he asked Allison, who worked at one of the Department of Agriculture labs, to collect tears from horses, cows, hens, ducks, and geese to see if there was lysozyme in them. Fleming also got the London Zoo to provide samples from fifty different species. In other tests, he located lysozyme in the eggs of the thrush, the moorhen, and the wagtail, as well as in parts of lupine, sunflowers, carnations, buttercup, elder, nettle, and candytuft; quite fittingly, he also found it in the milk of lactating women. He concluded that this substance might have something to do with protecting the body from bacteria that travel in the air because it showed up in most of the main doorways to the body—the nose, eyes, mouth, and respiratory tract.

Fleming was never able to isolate the active agent from the fluids, but he presumed that because it brought about a chemical change it was an enzyme. (Enzymes are cellular catalysts. For instance, it is the enzymes in laundry spray that break down the stains in clothes so they will wash out.) Eventually Wright named it lysozyme—a portmanteau word derived from *lysis*, in this case the ability to dissolve something else, and *enzyme*. Fleming had first thought he was dealing with what was then called a bacteriophage and is now called a virus, but because a virus soon replicates itself into billions of clones and an enzyme can't replicate, he revised his thinking. He did find that it destroyed about 75 percent of airborne bacteria and many other kinds as well. Unfortunately, lysozyme was effective only against harmless bacteria; fearsome strains of streptococci, staphylococci, and the bacteria that brought on tuberculosis and pneumonia were unfazed by it. Even so, while lysozyme was not an antibiotic of dramatic power, interest in its curious properties would have a direct role in the development of penicillin.

Fleming devoted considerable work to lysozyme in the years that followed his discovery. Between 1922 and 1932 he published eight papers about lysozyme, four of them before the end of 1924. Probably because it had no effect on anything that caused serious illness, the papers met with indifference for many years.

A scientist with a persuasive manner can capture the attention of his peers. Fleming was not persuasive. His limited skills as a writer and speaker contributed to this indifference. His papers are admirably brief and well organized, but they often lack precise experimental details. His reticence carried over to his public performances. His lectures to medical students were accompanied by clever practical demonstrations, but he was by every account a dreadful speaker; even though what he had to say was at least interesting and often impressive, it was offered more with self-deprecation than it was with conviction. One former student recalled that "his lectures were largely avoided by students" because his voice was scarcely audible, even to those in the front row. "I never heard Alexander Fleming raise his voice ever. He just had that low, rather monotonous delivery which meant that however exciting what he was talking about was to him, it didn't come across to the students."

These liabilities were painfully evident on an evening in December 1921 after Fleming presented a paper on lysozyme to the Medical Research Club. The club had been created in 1881, principally by Almroth Wright, as a forum for scientists to discuss current work and uncover further avenues of research. In spite of his failings as a conversationalist, Fleming was an amiable fellow, and he was a popular member of the club. Even so, when the chairman of the club asked for comments or questions after Fleming concluded his remarks, there was only silence. Perhaps no one fully heard what he had said, but it is also likely that his discovery seemed so obscure as to not warrant further interest.

Now seven years after discovering lysozyme in the clutter of his workbench, Fleming found another substance with microbial antagonism—penicillin—in even messier circumstances. He would say later that if he had been tidier or had had to work under the conditions of cleanliness of a pharmaceutical lab, he would never have discovered either.

Root-Bernstein's view is that Fleming was looking for lysozyme activity. He suggests that the penicillin mold indeed grew during a period of cold days but that Fleming didn't notice the plate until mid-September. In this scenario, Fleming then tested the mold for lysozyme activity and the results, as he shows in his published paper, were only mildly positive and thus he overlooked them. He put the plate on the stack in the Lysol tub and reexamined it when—later in the month than he recalled in 1944—Pryce stopped by. It was then that he noticed the weak activity and showed the plate to others in the lab, none of whom were particularly impressed.

"Not very novel," Root-Bernstein writes. "Not very impressive. Not even worth recording. Just another lysozyme experiment, with a mold this time."

Fleming's official biographer André Maurois noted that "Pryce had often seen old microbial colonies which for various reasons had dissolved. He thought that probably the mold was producing acids which were harmful to the staphylococci—no unusual occurrence." Pryce added that Fleming immediately put a bit of the mold in a test tube of broth to preserve it, but nothing is recorded.

After that, according to Root-Bernstein, Fleming cultured the mold, which took a couple of weeks. Around October 20, six weeks later than the usual time line, he grew the mold at room temperature for five days, then began a controlled experiment to see whether the mold was secreting lysozyme. He put it with bacteria known to be sensitive to it as well as with some of the *Staphylococcus* he had in abundance and incubated the bacteria. On October 30, he noted the results because they were quite stunning. The mold worked against a pathogen on which lysozyme has no effect. "Therefore," he recorded in his notebook, "mould culture contains a bacteriolytic substance for staphylococci."

"Now I ask you," Root-Bernstein writes, "if you had first observed this mold clearly dissolving staph cultures in early September . . . if you already had in your hands the beautiful plate everyone thinks is the original contamination—would you bother recording such a conclusion some six weeks later in the context of another experiment? I doubt it." Instead, he concludes, "the October 30 experiment is exactly what it seems to be within the context of the notebooks: the first penicillin experiment—the first recognition by Fleming that he's dealing with something unexpected and exciting."

Fleming's records from the end of October onward are more informative. Over the next months he conducted many experiments to learn more about penicillin. He asked his downstairs neighbor La Touche to identify the curious mold, and La Touche—wrongly, as it turned out—said it was *Penicillium rubrum*. (It would be more than two years before the error was discovered and the proper identification of a rare variant of *Penicillium notatum* was made.) Fleming also tried to determine if any of the thousands of known molds had the same power. He looked for samples on everything from old books and paintings to cheeses, breads, and jams. He even asked his friends at the Chelsea Arts Club for moldy old shoes they may have had about, which prompted a good deal of mirth.

The idea that mold could be a curative or an antibiotic was not a new one. Folk medicine in the early Greek and Roman societies and more recently in others as disparate as Ukraine and Mexico prescribed fungi, particularly mushrooms, and molds from bread and other items for the treatment of wounds and disease. Hippocrates found that fungi and especially yeast counter certain gynecological ailments, and Pliny the Elder devoted a chapter of *Historia Naturalis* to mushrooms as a remedy for *"rheumatismi."* (These astute observations lost currency during medieval times, when doctors favored such tonics as crocodile dung and eunuch's fat.) The Mayans treated ulcers and intestinal infections with a fungus known as *"cuxum,"* which grew on roasted green corn that was then left undisturbed for a period. Well into the twentieth century Ukrainian, Yugoslavian, and Greek peasants applied bread mold to wounds, feeling that it was more curative than manufactured drugs. The most novel fungal folk medicine appears in *Theatrum Botanicum* (1640) by John Parkinson, apothecary of London and king's herbarist.

Muscus ex cranio humano: "The Mosse upon dead mens sculles. . . . it should be taken from the sculles of those that have been hanged or executed for offences."

What seems to be the first recorded suggestion in a "modern" medical journal that a microorganism could have therapeutic value is in a letter in an 1852 issue of *The Lancet* describing the use of a tablespoon of yeast mixed with water and administered three times a day for the treatment of "troublesome boils," which, the author noted, "are equally as painful to bear as obstinate to cure, hardly yielding to any treatment by ordinary medical means. . . ."

Penicillium had long been a recognized type, and in 1876, the physicist and natural philosopher John Tyndall described the effects of it he had observed:

The mutton . . . gathered over it a thick blanket of *Penicillium* . . . [and] assumed a light brown colour, "as if by a faint admixture of clay"; but the infusion became transparent. The "clay" here was the slime of dead or dormant *Bacteria,* the cause of their quiescence being the blanket of *Penicillium.*

In every case where the mold was thick and coherent the *Bacteria* died, or became dormant, and fell to the bottom of the sediment. The growth of the mould and its effect on the *Bacteria* was very capricious. . . . The *Bacteria* which manufacture a green pigment appear to be uniformly victorious in their fight with the *Penicillium.* . . .

Tyndall described the characteristics of three different strains of *Penicillium* but seemed unaware that it was not the mold itself but rather a chemical substance produced by it that prevented the bacteria from growing.

The next and the most important intellectual step was taken in 1877 by Pasteur, who, with Jules-François Joubert, noticed that some airborne organisms stopped the growth of anthrax bacteria. Pasteur made a huge leap in scientific thinking when he deduced that this microbial warfare might fight disease, that it could be beneficial for one living thing to kill another.

That leap landed him at a spot with a hitherto unseen view. "In the inferior and vegetable species, still more than in the big animal and vegetable species," Pasteur wrote, prefacing one of his most quoted and profound observations, "life hinders life. A liquid invaded by an organized ferment, or by an aerobe, makes it difficult for an inferior organism to multiply. . . . These facts may, perhaps, justify the greatest hope from the therapeutic point of view."

Indeed they did. The use of life to hinder the life of organisms harmful to humans is a cornerstone of medicine as we know it.

Many stumbled upon penicillin; Fleming was the only one to look at what he tripped over. Among those who failed to examine what they saw was the Belgian scientist Dr. André Gratia and his associate Sara Dath. In the course of collecting and examining many molds and fungi at the Pasteur Institute outside Brussels in the 1920s, they came upon a petri dish of *Staphylococcus* colonized by a mold almost identical to the one Fleming noticed. Instead of culturing the mold, they simply noted its existence and effect. Once the marvelous nature of penicillin was finally understood, Gratia realized that he rather than

Fleming could have been the recipient of great fame and glory and never forgave himself for his lapse.

Fleming, however, worked on. After he found that none of the other molds he gathered produced the penicillin effect, he decided to delve deeper into the one that did and enlisted the help of his young but longtime assistant Stuart Craddock. Craddock had been looking into whether small doses of mercuric chloride (a colorless, odorless, but horrifically toxic compound) injected into microbes would weaken them and thus help phagocytes—the white blood cells that surround, kill, and digest cellular debris—do their work. "The only usable antiseptic," Fleming often reminded Craddock, "would be one which would arrest the growth of microbes without destroying the tissues." Such a substance, Fleming said, would transform the whole treatment of infections.

Fleming and Craddock soon made a large batch of broth from protein-rich bull's heart to feed the mold as it formed on the surface. As the mold grew, its antibiotic qualities mixed with the broth, but Fleming and Craddock quickly noticed that it was a transient guest; when the broth was left at room temperature, its antibacterial strength quickly diminished, which meant penicillin was very unstable. Tests showed that when stable, it was effective against some very tough bacterial customers. Beside *Streptococcus* and *Staphylococcus*, penicillin worked against the bacteria that cause pneumonia, gonorrhea, meningitis, and diphtheria. Typhoid, paratyphoid, and the influenza (or Pfeiffer's) bacillus, which Fleming had spent a good deal of time studying trying to find a cure for the common cold, were unaffected by the broth. Happily, penicillin, unlike carbolic acid, did not destroy the white blood cells' ability to eat bacteria and caused them no ill effects. It was also highly concentrated. Fleming and Craddock found that even when diluted to one part in eight hundred parts of water, penicillin still arrested bacteria. Penicillin had the look of the long-sought "perfect antiseptic."

Excited by these results, Fleming next performed a toxicity test, to see whether penicillin was poisonous; no antiseptic had passed such a test. He injected 20 cc's into a healthy rabbit. Penicillin showed itself to be no more toxic than the same quantity of broth. Half a cc injected into a healthy mouse also showed no toxicity. Constant irrigation of large infected surfaces in humans brought no toxic symptoms, and irrigation of eyes every hour for a day caused no irritation.

There was a severely limiting downside, however. An injection of broth into a rabbit's ear by Craddock at the end of March 1929 showed that penicillin's activity virtually ceased within thirty minutes, an indication that it would make a poor systemic medicine.

Scientists in later years would wonder why Fleming did not inject penicillin into a mouse made ill with staphylococcus, which would have been the obvious way to test its effectiveness as an antibiotic; such an experiment might have speeded the development of penicillin by a decade.

From his experience in working under Wright, Ronald Hare believed that Fleming ignored doing what most other scientists would have done "not because of any dislike of vivisection, but because the current doctrine was that infection of animals by injecting organisms was so artificial a proceeding that any lessons learned as a result would probably not be applicable to naturally acquired human infections. The causation and pathology of such infections were judged to be very different," an example of how far medicine has advanced in seventy-five years and a reminder that what is obvious in one era was not at all obvious in the one before it; indeed, it is precisely these leaps of knowledge that usher in new eras.

Fleming persisted. On January 9, 1929, he took a swab from Craddock's infected sinus to count the bacteria present, then put 1 cc of mold broth into the sinus; a swab taken three hours later showed that 99 percent of the bacteria were gone. It was an interesting result but not the basis for much celebration, because the broth contained so many contaminants. There was no hope that in its unpurified state penicillin could be a useful drug because those contaminants might cause anaphylactic shock, an often fatal reaction; anaphylactic shock is what kills people who are severely allergic to bee stings. Craddock then tried to cultivate penicillin in milk. After a week the milk had curdled and the juice had turned rather like Stilton cheese, which Craddock and another patient ate, to no effect.

Fleming now wanted to try the filtrate on an infected wound and asked doctors at the hospital to let him try it on a patient. They chose a woman who had slipped while leaving Paddington Station and fallen under a bus. Her leg was so damaged that it had to be amputated. Then septicemia had set in. Fleming put a dressing soaked in mold juice on the stump, but the unrefined broth was too weak to do any good. Fleming was not particularly surprised, because the juice was still so impure.

About this time he decided to name the substance discharged by the mold into the broth. "Mould juice" didn't have much of a ring to it. He thought penicillin was an enzyme but "penicillinzyme" was at least as bad as "mould juice." He thought *penicillin* from *penicillium* was as logical as *digitalin* from *digitalis*, because the suffix "-in" is found in such enzymes as trypsin and pepsin. Because Fleming had not isolated the active ingredient, in February 1929 he named the filtrate penicillin.

The questions surrounding penicillin were more chemical than biological, and Fleming needed a chemist to further his work. Unfortunately, there was no chemist on Wright's staff. The closest alternative was a newly qualified doctor with an amateur interest in chemistry, Frederick Ridley, who had helped Fleming try to purify lysozyme in 1926. Fleming asked him to work with Craddock, and Ridley agreed to do so. Because there was so little lab space, they set up shop in a narrow corridor outside the main lab; they constructed most of their apparatus from odds and ends lying around. None of the other scientists paid much attention to their work except when it was necessary to use the lavatory and they found their way to it blocked by these two large young men and their flasks of mold juice.

"Ridley," Craddock later recalled, "had sound and pretty advanced ideas about chemistry, but when it came to methods of extraction, we were driven back on the books. We read up a description of the classic method: using acetone, ether or alcohol as solvent, and evaporating the broth at a fairly low temperature, because we knew that great heat would destroy the substance; working in a vacuum. We knew very little when we began. We knew just a little bit more when we had finished."

They evaporated the broth by vacuum for fear that heat would make the penicillin disappear. The residue was a syrupy brown stuff rather like melted toffee. It was ten to fifty times stronger than the penicillin in the broth, but it needed to be purer still to be of use. Their goal was to make purified penicillin crystals. They could not inject penicillin still mixed with broth because the proteins from the broth would cause anaphylactic shock, bringing on difficulty in breathing and collapse of the blood veins.

Craddock added that he and Ridley were "full of hope when we started but as we went on, week after week, we could get nothing but this glutinous mass which . . . retained its power for about a week, but after a fortnight it became inert. . . . We had been so often discouraged. We thought we had got the thing. We put it in the refrigerator, only to find, after a week, that it had begun to vanish. Had an experienced chemist come on the scene, I think we could have got across that last hurdle. Then we could have published our results. But the expert did not materialize" and after a couple of months they abandoned their research and moved on to other jobs elsewhere. Fleming had not been involved in their work because he felt he was "a bacteriologist, not a chemist."

Despite these setbacks, Fleming remained intrigued with his find. Convinced that there was value in it, on February 13, 1929, he delivered a paper to the Medical Research Club entitled "A Medium for the Isolation of Pfeiffer's Bacillus" (presumably about using penicillin as a means of inhibiting a particular bacterium in cultures). The evening was a replay of his 1921 paper on lysozyme.

"He was very shy, and excessively modest in his presentation," Henry Dale, a leading physiologist who was then chairman of the club and who would go on to become one of the most powerful and influential British scientists of his time, told Maurois in the late 1950s. "He gave it in a half-hearted sort of way, shrugging his shoulders as though he were deprecating the importance of what he had said." When he finished, he remained at the podium to answer any questions; once again there were none, not even a polite query out of kindness. Perhaps his listeners simply regarded this as another of Fleming's mildly interesting but not particularly useful finds; Pfeiffer's bacillus was not currently in vogue with researchers. Or perhaps once again his delivery had been so quiet and unexpressive that no one was able to properly hear what he said and thus grasp the importance of what was inferred. Whatever the cause, the audience soon gathered themselves. The next paper, "On the Nature of the Lesion in Generalized Vaccinia," enthralled them.

Dale, reminiscing a generation after the fact and at the height of Fleming's fame, put the best spin he could on the reaction of those present, as if to explain why he and his fellows could not possibly have failed to comprehend one of the seminal discoveries of the century. Despite Fleming's verbal presentation, "All the same the elegance and beauty of his observations made a great impression." If it was true, it was an impression they failed to convey to Fleming, who nearly twenty-five years after the event still referred to the ensuing silence as "that frightful moment."

Undeterred—even bravely—in May, Fleming submitted a paper entitled "On the Antibacterial Action of Cultures of a Penicillium with Special Reference to Their Use in the Isolation of B. Influenzae" to the *British Journal of Experimental Pathology*. In keeping with the custom of the Inoculation Department, he first showed the paper to Wright so that its publication would be authorized by him. Wright objected to the eighth of Fleming's ten summarized observations about penicillin: "It is suggested that it may be an efficient antiseptic for application to, or injection into, areas affected with penicillin-sensitive microbes." To Wright, this was near heresy. He was convinced that antiseptics were ineffectual and even counterproductive and that only the body's natural defenses—and vaccines that imitated them—were curative. Fleming held his ground and the passage appeared as written when the paper was published the next month.

Because Fleming used words with an economy that bordered on miserly, his paper is about as far from a model of scientific discourse as his presentation to the Medical Research Club was of compelling rhetoric. It sets out what he did and what he learned but so much of exactly how he did what he did is omitted that it is not possible to accurately repeat his experiment. Hare believed this was because unlike most scientists, for whom the results of experiments are paramount, what mattered most to Fleming was "not the recording of his experiments but . . . the actual performance of the experiment that he loved."

Fleming would work fitfully on penicillin until 1935, although a second paper published in 1932 was really the end of his active interest, which lasted longer than anyone else's. His 1929 paper went scarcely noticed for ten years. Eventually that changed. Because the paper is the starting point of the antibiotic revolution, despite its flaws it has come to be regarded as one of the most important medical papers ever written.

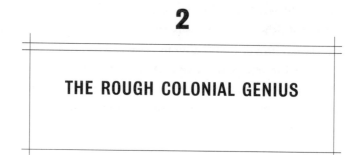

2

THE ROUGH COLONIAL GENIUS

One of the editors of the *British Journal of Experimental Pathology* when it published Fleming's paper on penicillin in 1929 was Howard Walter Florey, an Australian who came to Oxford in 1922 as a Rhodes scholar. He spoke the same language as his fellow students, but in accent and manner he was clearly from away, something he made no effort to hide and sometimes even enjoyed. He wrote with amusement to a friend in Australia that at a tea party not long after his arrival, "I endeavoured to look like the hardened criminal of the bush everyone expected." They didn't expect it for long. Florey's ambition, his hard work, and his talent quickly made him prominent in British scientific research.

In the 1880s his father, Joseph, emigrated with his wife and two young daughters from England to Adelaide, where he established what became a prosperous boot-making business. He remarried after his first wife died from tuberculosis; two more daughters followed. The last child and only son, Howard, was born on September 24, 1898. He was immediately subject to the adoration of his sisters and parents, who dressed him in prissy clothes reminiscent of Thomas Gainsborough's *Blue Boy* and left his hair to grow below his shoulders in a curly cascade until after his eighth birthday.

The family first lived in a modest cottage about ten miles outside Adelaide, but success soon brought a large house in a wealthy enclave. Howard attended a local private school where he was given the nick-

name "Floss" or "Flos," which stuck for the remainder of his life; his
son Charles has always understood that it came from the Latin for
flower, *"flos"* or *"flor."* In 1911, he entered fashionable St. Peter's
Collegiate School, in Adelaide. Modeled on the English public schools,
it was one of the best in the country. However, there would be no
confusion in picking a St. Peter's student from, say, an Etonian. These
were Australian boys, by nature of their culture independent, informal,
and unpretentious. While on a Rockefeller Foundation fellowship in
the United States when he was twenty-seven, Florey was affectionately
described as "a rough colonial genius."

Science captivated him, though he missed some details. When he
was twelve, he enthusiastically announced to his sister Hilda, the only
female medical student in her class at Adelaide University, that he
wanted to be a researcher. Amused, she said, "Oh, you'd like to be a
sort of Pasteur?" He had no idea what she meant.

Florey won a school prize in chemistry in his first year. Although
by his own admission he was no good at mathematics, and despite
bouts of pneumonia in 1912 and 1914 and recurrent severe bronchitis,
he finished first in his class in physics and chemistry every year
thereafter. He showed no interest in entering his father's business, but
the headmaster of St. Peter's dashed his hopes for becoming a chemist
by saying there was no future for one in Australia. Although that was
not completely true, Florey turned to medicine because, he later said,
"it was a reasonable thing to do," a decision perhaps made easier by
the knowledge that his liabilities in math would limit his abilities as a
physicist.

By the time Howard entered Adelaide University Medical School in
March 1916, his father's health was failing. So was his business, which
had sold shares to the public in 1912 and been put in the care of a
manager whose incompetent and even dishonest management sped
them down the road to ruin. Joseph was forced to mortgage all his
property to save the family from total financial collapse. Fortunately,
at the end of Howard's final term at St. Peter's, he won a notable
prize as well as a state scholarship to pay all his medical school tuition
and fees.

Florey was one of only two dozen students in the medical school, which was generally considered not to be the equal of those in England or America. Florey said later, "The teaching of physiology was hardly worth considering. Anatomy was quite good, biochemistry had hardly started." The school was geared to turning out practitioners of medicine rather than researchers; students were told, "It is far better for you to learn what is in your books. It is not for you to question." Florey turned to self-reliance in learning; he and his classmates talked in groups about physiology and other subjects to boost their knowledge. Florey's rigor in studying kept him at the top of his class.

When he was at ease he was engaging and popular, but he approached neither work nor play with half measures. A determined and talented athlete, he was never a social one. At tennis he focused not only on winning but also on winning convincingly, and he often offended those with whom he played. He upbraided partners for missing shots or for relaxing even when it was clear the match was won, and he glared across the net at opponents, men and women alike. He was almost genetically incapable of giving direct praise, to others or to himself, and his backhanded compliments could be especially unsettling to those who did not know he lauded their good work behind their backs.

Howard's fiery personality was contrasted by his almost startling good looks. Though he was only about five-foot-seven, his lean face, his eyes at once piercing and soulful, and his swept-back hair neatly parted in the middle combined to give him an arresting presence.

In September 1918, Joseph died of a heart attack, age sixty-one. His company soon died as well. Joseph's shares were worthless, and all that saved the Floreys from complete insolvency was his wife Bertha's canny earlier conversion of her own common shares to preferred ones. In 1920, the family moved into a small bungalow similar to the one in which Howard was born.

In this difficult time Howard had to make a difficult decision about his future. He was by now convinced that his life's work lay in medical research rather than in clinical medicine, but "there were no opportunities in the sort of things I was beginning to get interested in, physiology, for example. . . . The universities and the medical schools and the science departments were not well equipped and hadn't the background for research, and of course this colored my life." He would have to go elsewhere to study and leave the family to fend for itself. He weighed whether to take an inferior medical job in Adelaide, which would bring in cash to help support his mother and sisters, or to apply for a Rhodes scholarship, which would pay for three years' study and provide endless opportunity at Oxford but no financial help at home. With considerable mixed feelings, he applied for the scholarship. His abilities as a student and as an athlete (besides tennis he played cricket and football), his work on the Adelaide Medical Students Society *Review* and the *Adelaide University Magazine*, and the high recommendations of his teachers won him the Rhodes. In 1921, he finished first in his medical examinations and was graduated from Adelaide University.

It was in his capacity as editor of the *Review* that Howard met Ethel Hayter Reed, a bank manager's daughter and one of the few female medical students. She was three years behind him in her studies but far ahead of him socially. Attractive, obviously intelligent, and popular, she was possessed of an ambition that burned as bright as his own. Howard was taken by her and, in January 1920, used the ruse of asking her to write an article for the *Review* entitled "Women in Medicine" to get to know her better. It worked. Over the next two years they saw a good deal of each other, with interruptions for Ethel's convalescence from two bouts of pleurisy, a painful inflammation of the lungs. Before long, Howard fell in love with her, though neither was certain of their future together. She was twenty-one and recuperating in the mountains from her second round of pleurisy when he wrote to her just before he sailed for England.

"You're the only person, male or female, to whom I can go down to bedrock, or very near it anyway," he told her. He also said how sad he was to leave his family. "I'm dreading the family 'goodbye' tomorrow. I shan't see my mother again, probably, and I've been a beast—that's the rub. If a chap could dispense with a conscience, or be like Elija and push off in a chariot these things wouldn't worry one."

He left Australia—for good, he thought—at the height of the Australian summer in December 1921 and worked his way to England as a ship's surgeon, arriving in wintry Oxford in January 1922. His choice to become a student at Magdalen College put him in one of the most prestigious as well as one of the most class conscious of the university's colleges. Florey's nationality, his schooling, and his financial status all assured indifferent treatment by his fellow students, but it seems not to have mattered to him; he was willing to settle instead for the admiration of his professors. Being Australian, he felt "one could get away with any sort of gaucheries" if so desired, but he also realized that at Oxford "if you show any signs of being good at all, you get encouraged" by the professors and tutors. He made an immediate impression on the secretary of the Rhodes Trust, who wrote that Florey was a "first-rate man—ranks with our best."

Florey also impressed John Fulton, an American Rhodes scholar with whom he shared a First Class in the Honours School of Physiology in 1923. "I don't quite know how it happened—all the others couldn't know much," he wrote to Ethel. "As a point of fact and I may as well say so, I'm rather pleased. There were 64 for the show and only 5 Firsts."

In today's lexicon, it would be said that Florey had poor social skills and that he kept himself at a distance from others. For example, Fulton seems the only person outside Florey's immediate family whom he ever called by his first name; the two maintained a close correspondence throughout their lives. Robert Webb, with whom he later formed a friendship at Cambridge that would last more than forty years, always called Florey by his family nickname, "Floss," but was called "Webb" in return. This standoffishness was evident not only in address but also in Florey's unwillingness or inability to mingle, and it denied him other friendships.

"I can see myself developing into a rather nasty product," he wrote to Ethel at the end of 1923. "I'm that most damnably lonely I don't know what to do, sometimes. I'm not complaining against anyone or anything—people in Oxford have been exceedingly decent to me . . . but the fact is I haven't really got a friend as I conceive the term, and am quite incapable of having one." Earlier he had written, "Happiness comes from within . . . I don't think anyone can be happy in any one period. I'm talking about myself, as usual. I've got opportunities most chaps would give a lot for and yet I'm not satisfied. It's a frightfully lonely business living among strangers."

To Webb, Florey was unconcerned about popularity. "I think he just . . . felt himself different from people around him. He knew he could work for what he wanted to achieve and go on longer than others."

Most notably for his future, Florey caught the attention of Sir Charles Sherrington, the Oxford Professor of Physiology. He would share the Nobel Prize for physiology or medicine in 1932 for discoveries regarding the functions of neurons. Sherrington's 1904 book, *The Integrative Action of the Nervous System*, brought neurophysiology into the modern age. He coined the terms *neuron* (the nerve cell) and *synapse* (the point at which the nerve impulse is transmitted from one nerve cell to another), and his work on nerve function has been a prime influence on the development of brain surgery and the treatment of paralysis, atrophy, and other nervous disorders. He is as well the namesake of Sherrington's law, which states that when one set of muscles is stimulated, muscles opposing the action are simultaneously inhibited. In 1923, Sherrington was also president of the Royal Society, the most distinguished scientific organization in Britain and one of the two or three most prominent in the world.

Sherrington, whose nickname was "Sherry" or "Sherrie" and who by every account was as kind as he was brilliant, appreciated Florey's tenacity to take on problems of his own initiative. A colleague of Florey's for many decades says that Sherrington was "perhaps the only man that the mature Florey looked up to." At Sherrington's suggestion Florey did what turned out to be seminal work on the vessels of a cat's brain when he observed that unlike some arteries in the body, these were insensitive to adrenaline. "I've had a cat with a glass window in its head running round the lab, which amused me greatly," he wrote to Ethel.

Sherrington was known to look out for students from abroad, but his treatment of Florey was almost paternal. In 1923, Sherrington began a correspondence with Florey that traces Florey's rapid rise as a scientist of distinction. The first commends Florey "for the excellent work you have done" and invites him to come and work in his lab (John Fulton also worked there with him). Three years later, Sherrington writes with evident joy after Florey received another of the many prizes he would win, "There have been such a series of congratulating events in regard to you that my pen is running out." By 1929, congratulations have been replaced by requests for advice on revisions in his then widely used text *Mammalian Physiology: A Course of Practical Exercises.*

As a partial result of Sherrington's enthusiasm for Florey and his work, in 1923, Florey was awarded the prestigious John Lucas Walker Studentship at Cambridge, which paid £300 per year and an additional £200 for apparatus, a living wage but not more. Sherrington had convinced him that it was time for someone with a background in physiology, the study of the processes and function of the human body, to do experimental work in pathology, the study of the characteristics, causes, and effects of disease in the body.

"The thing that tickles my fancy is that it is pathology and I don't know any," he wrote to Ethel. "However they think I know some physiology and rather like my idea (not mine really, of course!) of doing pathological physiology." The idea, of course, was Sherrington's, who also felt that the studentship—which had been an open competition to any student in Britain—was the best avenue for a career in experimental medicine.

It was a decisive moment in Florey's career. The award signaled to the scientific community that he was a young man of consequence, and Florey recognized his heightened status. "I couldn't possibly get a better launching into experimental medicine," he told Ethel. "It means if I do any good at all that I'll get a decent lectureship, and possibly in a few years' time a professorship. (Altogether too rosy probably but I feel a bit buoyed up by it.)"

At Cambridge Florey joined Gonville and Caius College ("Gonville is never talked about except officially," he told Ethel in another letter, "—it's 'Caius' and 'Caius' is pronounced 'keys' "), where he was taken under the wing of Dr. Henry Roy Dean, a highly regarded and influential immunologist who believed in an experimental approach to science and who had recently been made the Professor of Pathology. Florey impressed Dean with his intelligence and capability and perhaps flattered him with his admiration. Florey's English biographer, Gwyn Macfarlane, writes that he "deeply respected the scientific leaders of his day—in fact, he was frankly dazzled by them. They, in their turn, responded with a personal interest in this ebullient young Australian."

Before he joined Dean, Florey spent the summer of 1924 on the ship *Polar Bjorn* as the medical officer of the Oxford University Arctic Expedition to Spitsbergen to explore and study the geology and natural history of the largely glacial arctic islands. On his return, Florey was beset by attacks of indigestion. He told Ethel he didn't know whether it was appendix trouble or a gastric ulcer or simply dyspepsia. His doctor diagnosed achlorhydria, a lack of the normal hydrochloric acid in the stomach. Florey became adept at inserting a tube down his throat and into his stomach to gather stomach mucus or insert medicine to aid his dyspepsia. He wrote to Ethel, "What I'm most proud of is I can swallow a stomach tube almost like breakfast now and have a jolly time moving bicarbonate in and out."

Beginning at Cambridge and continuing for the rest of his career, mucous secretion was a major topic of Florey's work, and of his contributions to science. His reaction to his illness illuminates his scientific interests. Professor Sir Henry Harris, an Australian who worked under Florey at Oxford and who succeeded him as Professor of Pathology when he retired in 1963, noted in his memoir, *The Balance of Probabilities*, that virtually all of Florey's research stemmed from diseases that afflicted him or members of his family.

His lifelong interest in the physiology and pathology of the intestinal tract arose from problems he had with his own. As a young man at Cambridge he had suffered from severe dyspepsia, which had been misdiagnosed as achlorhydria. . . . It appears that for a while he had been advised to take hydrochloric acid with his meals. ("Didn't do anything but rot my teeth, Harris.") By the time I knew him, he did not seem to have anything wrong with his stomach, but he was often much concerned with his bowels. ("You don't know what pleasure it can be to make a formed stool, Harris.") To what extent all this suffering had its origin in nervous tension can now be only a matter of conjecture, but as far as his own bodily functions were concerned Florey was certainly a very introspective man.

Harris added,

> No interpretation of the last 20 years of Florey's life can be other than superficial if it does not take into account that during the whole of this period he was subject to recurrent bouts of angina. The emergence of his interest in arteriosclerosis [a hardening of the walls of the arteries], and quite specifically arteriosclerosis of the coronary arteries, was prompted by his own cardiac pain.

At Cambridge, Florey immediately justified the faith that Sherrington and Dean had placed in him. In his first year, he had four papers published in influential journals, two of them on cerebral circulation. But as at Oxford, his academic and scientific successes with his professors were offset by his manner with his peers. One of his research collaborators later wrote to Florey's Australian biographer, Lennard Bickel:

> Florey was not an easy personality. His drive and ambition were manifest from the day he arrived. A great fire seemed to burn within him, and his many-sided character was never concealed. We could all see the power in him and wondered whether he would ever find the right outlets for his greatness. This was the beginning of a remarkable career and he was very determined to succeed. He could be ruthless and selfish; on the other hand, he could show kindliness, a warm humanity, and, at times, sentiment and a sense of humour. He displayed utter integrity and he was scathing of humbug and pretence. His attitude was always—"You must take me as you find me." But, to cope with him at times, you had to do battle, to raise your voice as high as his and never let him shout you down. You had to raise your pitch to his but if you insisted on your right he was always, in the end, very fair. I must say that at times, he went out of his way to cut people down to size with some very destructive criticism. But I must also say that in the years I knew him he did not once utter a word of praise about himself.

Florey was eager to follow whatever career prospect he could. In 1922, he spent three months in clinics in Vienna—he wrote to Ethel that he hoped to meet Freud—and in 1923 spent a month in Copenhagen learning new techniques in investigating capillaries. In 1925, at the end of his first year at Cambridge and in further affirmation of his increasing prestige, Florey was awarded a Rockefeller Foundation fellowship to go to the United States to study techniques of microdissection—the cutting and examination of tiny veins or bits of tissue. Over a period of ten months ending in May 1926, he studied in university labs in New York City, in Chicago, and, most important, at the University of Pennsylvania in Philadelphia with Dr. Alfred Newton Richards, a prominent physiologist who would later become president of the National Academy of Sciences. Richards was taken by the young man he called "a rough colonial genius"; fifteen years later this good relationship would be of inestimable value to Florey and to the world.

In the four years since leaving Adelaide, Howard wrote over 130 letters to Ethel, telling her of his progress and plans. They reveal that Howard was a wild romantic in his view of Ethel, while Ethel, willing to be wooed, was much more hardheaded and pragmatic. The popular twenty-one-year-old girl he had left behind suffered numerous illnesses, was beset by a disease that attacks the middle ear, causing ever-increasing deafness, and by 1925 was a toughened new doctor—she was the only woman in her class to complete medical school—fascinated by medicine and coming to terms with her own ambitions. She held an internship at Adelaide Children's Hospital and had a good medical career ahead of her there but no prospects in England. While Howard was in America she wrote,

> I am quite prepared to give the whole thing up when I marry you. But in return I must feel absolutely certain of your unreserved, and entire love for the whole of my life.
>
> I thought I was certain but your last letter shows me how little you know the real me. You still seem to think I ought to be some sort of inhuman angel instead of a quite typical modern girl with a terrific lot of weaknesses and a fair amount of intelligence and attractiveness. . . .

I am giving up everything else I've got for you Floss—that ought to
be proof enough that I love you. . . .

Much of this was ignored by Howard, who was desperate for her
to come to the United States and marry him. For a couple of years
she was generally willing but also racked by uncertainty. Several times
she said she would come, only to say in the next letter that she
couldn't. (It often took two or three months for a letter to cross the
ocean and its answer to sail back.) In his loneliness Howard had ide-
alized Ethel, and though he was unaware of that, she wasn't.

I've told you time and time again that I was not by any means the
perfect person you imagined me. . . .

If you don't think I'm worth your love Floss well—I'll just retire
behind the screens. I would quite agree with you. I've often wondered
what it was in me that made you love me. But I suppose I must have
forgotten that you endowed me with all the virtues you thought a
woman ought to possess and so fell in love with a false image. . . .

It does seem most important that we should have a time to get to
know each other better doesn't it?

Their reunion on Howard's birthday in September 1926 was not
as joyous as either anticipated; reality is often a poor reflection of
fantasy. Still, the next month they were wed in Trinity Church, Paddington, not far from St. Mary's Hospital. Several months later Howard and Ethel moved to Cambridge, where he was now Huddersfield
Lecturer in Special Pathology. He taught physiology and performed
research in pathology, was elected an official fellow of Gonville and
Caius College, and became director of medical studies. He was able
to move back into the same lab he had used before going to the United
States, but his old technician was unwilling to work for him; Florey,
he said, was far too demanding.

In his stead, Florey found fourteen-year-old James Kent sweeping
out the lab when he arrived to work his first morning. Florey took to
him immediately, and Kent, though he had been warned about Florey's penchant for driving his assistant, was unconcerned about how

much work he would have to do. He wanted to be a vet, and, when Florey asked if he liked working with animals, he was enthusiastic in his response. They would work together for forty years.

The richness of Howard's work was a sharp counterpoint to Ethel's, who instead of being a doctor was now a doctor's wife. In their years of correspondence, he often talked about their doing research together—they might have been like Pierre and Marie Curie— but once again the event did not match the anticipation. His experiments often required many hours of precise surgery, and a single misstep could ruin the work. Kent came to know his method and anticipate his needs, but Ethel's deafness led to misunderstandings of what instrument he asked for or what he wanted her to do, and when an experiment went wrong because of her errors, he was as ruthless with her as he was with any hapless assistant. As Macfarlane puts it, Howard's work "became a barrier rather than a bond. Since Ethel could not share it she came to resent it."

Despite these battles between two ambitious people, one leaping from success to success, the other trying only to find a foothold for her professional self-regard, there was also affection, at least for a while. Their daughter, Paquita Mary Joanna, alternatively abbreviated "Paq" or "Park," was born in 1929. Their son, Charles, followed in 1934, named in honor of Charles Sherrington and given the nickname "Egbert"; as time passed he became "Eg," then "Bertie." But by then, the marriage had soured so terribly that they hardly spoke; most communication was through notes left on a table. One day instead of a note, Howard found a detailed accounting of Ethel's grievances. It no longer exists, but her complaints are evident by Howard's fifteen-page handwritten point-by-point response, folded in an envelope addressed "Mrs. H. W. Florey."

My dear Girl,
Memorandum for memorandum. I have read yours with the closest attention and have gathered a number of impressions from it and made a number of resolutions as a result of it. Firstly let me say at once that I am now very sorry for many of the things I have said to you and I quite appreciate the many directions in which my conduct can be

improved. As I am now getting older I trust that I can move in a more placid direction and my best efforts will be directed to that. Nevertheless since you say I will never discuss anything with you I think perhaps I had better do so as you invite the opportunity. One thing which astonished me greatly was to learn that "for nearly eight years of my married life I have loved you dearly and deeply." You must pardon my astonishment and really accept my statement that I have perhaps a far higher admiration for "love" than you are inclined to give me credit for. . . .

He goes on to recount how poorly she treated him in writing letters from Australia, often delaying a response so long that it missed the boat for England, thus adding weeks more to his receiving it, and her cool greeting when she finally came. Ethel had stayed up late on the ship to reject a suitor and "yawned in my face," and on other occasions went to the theater with men friends she had met on the trip, leaving Howard alone at the rooming house she stayed in before they were married and the landlady "astonished."

It astonishes you perhaps that I have any feelings. Nevertheless I thought all would be well and that the things were not so serious as I thought. At great inconvenience we lived in Surrey where I was struck with horror when I realized how sick you were. You may say and honestly believe that you came at the time you did for love of me but unfortunately it then appeared to me that you had handed on your rather battered body to me after insisting on doing not only your general hospital work but also the Children's. It is all very well to tell me now of the brilliant career you had in front of you but you have evidently forgotten that you told me in those far off days that you thought your health would have precluded a very active medical life. You may not think so now but you did then nevertheless. . . .

Very soon after we were married you blandly informed me that if you didn't like married life you were going back to Australia. A nice conversational opening, and surely something to have told me *before* marriage. . . . As the result of these things and many trivialities I unfortunately did not realize you had any real affection for me. My disappointment was and is and always will be immense that you are even now not strong enough to share my pleasures as would a normal woman. . . . You must realize that you are not a physically normal woman—I refer to your deafness. It is a tragedy for you. I am fully aware of that but what you don't realize is that this tragedy extends in ever widening circles. You must accept my statement as true that to talk to a deaf person for long periods of time is very exhausting and it may be exasperating when one is accused of making statements when one knows that it is entirely your misapprehension which is to blame. . . .

So much for general considerations which I have sketched for your enlightenment. In spite of your devastating conduct and my very bad reactions there have been times when we have been quite tolerably happy and I see no reason why we shouldn't again reach such a desirable state. . . .

Howard proposed an allowance per quarter for personal needs, children, and housekeeping. "I want you to be quite clear that I do not expect you to provide me with any luxuries and all I ask is that any simple food you give me should be reasonably well cooked. If you cannot afford to buy fruit I shall not grumble." He also said that he would undertake all expenses for the children's education. Divorce, however, was not an option.

[A]s you have been injudicious enough to mention "legal separation" let me say that this would involve splitting the children between us. From their point of view this would be lamentable. . . . Although neither of us have got all we expected from our marriage there is still a good deal left which with a little good will can make more. Let us try. . . .

Sexual relations: If we are to make a real effort at reconciliation I think it is quite clear that we must live together sexually. If not it would be a constant source of irritation between us. I am really quite anxious to do this and I deeply regret the misunderstandings which have grown up during your pregnancy. . . . Nevertheless, anxious as I am that we should resume our previous relationship, my elephantine hide has been moderately deeply incised by your suggestion as to the manner in which you would permit me to use your body. I regard it as obscene and I particularly resent it as, to my knowledge, I have always been most solicitous and never forced myself on you when you were definitely averse. Surely you know I wouldn't dream of such a thing? However . . . if you can think to come to me again it is obvious that you must make it abundantly clear that you do so from choice and that I am not intimidating you.

Lunch: This has been a perennial source of trouble. In future all I ask for is a boiled egg when I come in, some bread, butter, milk and soda water. Surely you can give me this little . . . and not greet me with that look of baffled irritation which has become so painfully familiar. . . .

I make a few suggestions:

1. Realize your deafness is a handicap to others as well as yourself. Wear your earphones whenever possible.

2. Do not get angry unless you are *sure* you have heard aright.

3. Try to avoid picking your nose in my presence.

4. Wash your hair more often and by the introduction of a suitable amount of scent improve to smell. I know my breath smells frequently and perhaps you will think less badly of me if I tell you that I avoid coming too near you when I know this is the case.

5. Don't nag at me. Perhaps other ways will occur to you of being patient with my peculiarities.

Let us both resolve to do our utmost to heal the breech which has grown up and I am sure we will be successful. Now that we know some at least of the reasons for one another's discontents it may be easier for us to be forgiving and charitable.

Whatever his failures at home, Florey continually was regarded as a man with a bright future, and, by 1931, he was ready to move on to a professorship. When the chair of Professor of Pathology at Sheffield University opened, Florey applied. He was not an obvious choice, at least to traditionalists; one prominent pathologist is said to have looked at the list of candidates and announced, "There is no pathologist called Florey."

Strictly speaking, he was correct; Florey had never done a human autopsy (just as Fleming, a qualified surgeon, had never performed an operation). But forward-looking scientists saw the combination of physiology and pathology as the path of the future in the field, and two of those scientists were on the Sheffield selection committee. One was J. B. Lathes, the Professor of Physiology, who shared Sherrington's views on this, and the other was Edward Mellanby, the Professor of Pharmacology, whose work on rickets helped lead to the discovery of vitamin D. The two men often worked together and were considered the most outstanding scientists at the university. Florey won his new position in December. His passion helped seal his appointment. Florey later said that his electors gave him only one instruction: "We don't care what you do as long as you make a mess in this laboratory, it's been too clean for a number of years."

What small amount of work was done on penicillin in the early 1930s went mostly in a circle. In 1932, Harold Raistrick, who taught at the School of Tropical Medicine and Hygiene, was the first professional biochemist to try to purify it, from a sample sent him by Fleming. With his assistant Dr. P. W. Clutterbuck and bacteriologist Dr. R. Lovell, Raistrick duplicated most of Fleming's observations and generally followed the rocky trail of Ridley and Craddock, who had not published the results of their work. They all arrived at about the same dead end. Raistrick and his colleagues did, however, find that a synthetic growth medium of glucose in water with sodium, potassium, manganese, and iron was easier to use than the chemically complicated meat-digest broth made from bull's heart that Fleming, Craddock, and Ridley used. They found that penicillin is more stable in an acid solution and that impurities such as its yellow pigment could be eliminated with sulfuric acid. They also found that the active ingredient of penicillin could be extracted from the broth with alcohol and that it was soluble in acidified ether. But as penicillin in ether is useless as a medicine, and as there was no way they could find to extract it from the solvent without destroying it, there was no point in going on, especially since penicillin was yet to be seen to have any clinical use. Raistrick and his coresearchers published their results in the *British Medical Journal* in 1932 and then moved on to other things.

Fleming came to regret what he saw as a missed opportunity. In 1946, after penicillin was widely available, Fleming wrote to Florey that had he and Raistrick collaborated in the 1930s, they might have made better progress together than they did singly. It was "a pity" that they didn't, and he offered a rationale.

"In those days I was working in an immunological laboratory with a chief [Wright] whose sole interest was immunology. Antibiotics for me was rather a side line and when Raistrick published his paper showing that the concentration of penicillin was not quite successful even in the hands of an expert chemist, I'm afraid I got discouraged about that problem."

Others dabbled with penicillin, with little more success. In 1935, Dr. Cecil G. Paine, a former student at St. Mary's with Fleming and now a member of Florey's department in Sheffield, made some progress with mold juice from one of Fleming's cultures. Irrigation with his broth cured two babies born with gonorrheal eye infections and another case of staphylococcal conjunctivitis. His most dramatic success was with a patient whose right eye had been stabbed by debris in an accident. The bacteria that cause pneumonia settled in, making it impossible to operate. Two days of bathing the eye with the broth cleared the infection enough to remove the object, and the eye was saved. This treatment was interesting—and it did save an eye—but it led nowhere new scientifically. As it had with Fleming, the mold quickly lost its potency, making it a poor candidate for a useful drug. Paine later described the work as "uniformly disappointing." Moreover, because there was no biochemist available to work on the problem, there was little chance of any more success than Raistrick had. Penicillin remained an interesting novelty.

Then came a new discovery. The introduction of sulfa drugs in 1935 shoved aside any residual enthusiasm there may have been for penicillin. Paul Ehrlich's success with Salvarsan had encouraged researchers at the I. G. Farbenindustrie subsidiary Bayer pharmaceutical company, near Düsseldorf, to look for other chemical compounds that kill bacteria.

The hope that chemicals had medical potential became a serious possibility in 1856, when William Perkin invented the first artificial dye, mauve. It led to a rainbow of colors for clothes, made chemistry more practical, affected the development of explosives, and changed medicine. Before making his famous "606," Ehrlich showed that the bloodstream transported injected methylene blue dye and that the dye broke into fine particles before it entered the cells, staining them; "606" used a dye to alter the chemical structure of disease-causing microbes that caused syphilis.

Some dyes attach so firmly to proteins in fibers that they are impervious to cleaning or fading and Bayer's Gerhard Domagk reasoned that many of them might also attach to proteins in bacteria, inhibiting their effectiveness or even killing them. In 1932, Domagk, who had tested hundreds of compounds on infected animals, discovered that an orange-red dye called sulfamidochrysoidine with the trade name Prontosil protected mice from streptococcal infections. He worked in secret for the next three years and then published a short account of his results in 1935.

Prontosil was hard to come by for doctors eager to work with it themselves, most likely because Bayer kept the supply limited while looking for a way to patent the active ingredient. Leonard Colebrook, Fleming's colleague in testing Salvarsan, finally obtained some and found it was remarkably powerful against puerperal fever, a staphylococcal infection that attacked about 1 percent of new mothers and had a 25 percent mortality rate. Prontosil proved effective against meningitis and gonorrhea, too, but the dye also turned the patient's skin bright red. Researchers at the Pasteur Institute in Paris soon discovered that a substance in Prontosil called aminobenzenesulphonamide, soon named sulfanilamide, was the actual antibacterial agent and that it had the added value of not changing coloration. It is likely that Domagk already knew this but did not share the information because of Bayer's patenting concerns.

Hundreds of thousands of lives were saved by the group of medications called sulfonamides. However, the so-called wonder drug was not completely wondrous. It was ineffective in the presence of pus, and the heavy doses required caused rashes, vomiting, and kidney damage. Even so, it was proof again that chemotherapeutic compounds worked and that antibacterial agents put into the circulating blood could have a powerful curative effect.

Soon after the announcement of Prontosil, Fleming transferred his interest to sulfa drugs, but he kept a culture of penicillin going in his lab because "mould broth" was useful for cleansing petri dishes of unwanted bacteria during experiments. His discovery had come full circle. He had found penicillin as a contaminant in a petri dish. Now he was using it to decontaminate petri dishes.

During Florey's years at Sheffield, he hoped in vain to find the funding to pay the salary for a full-time biochemist to join in his investigations into mucus, lysozyme, tetanus, the lymphatic vessels, and gastrointestinal secretion. This work resulted in a dozen published papers in four years. At Sheffield, Florey's usual scientific success was accompanied by relatively better relations with his peers than he had at Oxford or Cambridge, in part because Yorkshire is the seat of plain speaking in England and thus suited Florey perfectly. "I have never met an educated man whose conversation stayed so close to the ground," Henry Harris says of Florey. "It was as if he deliberately shunned subtle or polished speech."

This, however, was hardly reason for Florey to spend his career in Sheffield. There was a prize professorship he longed for, and the opportunity to have it came sooner than anyone could imagine.

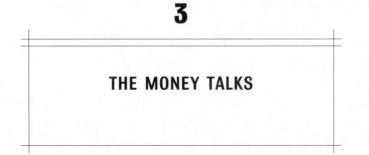

3

THE MONEY TALKS

The job that Florey had his eye on was the Chair of Pathology at Oxford University. Science was the greatest financial beneficiary at Oxford in the first years following the end of World War I, and one of its greatest benefactors was the estate of Sir William Dunn, whose trustees gave £100,000 to build and equip a school of pathology. Unfortunately Georges Dreyer, the Professor of Pathology, did not also secure an endowment to run it.

Dunn, a Scot who made his fortune in South Africa and died in 1912, left £1 million to promote a variety of causes, among them the advancement of Christianity and the alleviation of human suffering. Dreyer meticulously oversaw every detail of the construction and outfitting of the three-story Queen Anne–style Sir William Dunn School of Pathology. It abuts the University Parks, the hundreds of spectacular acres of grass, trees, a cricket pitch, and occasional bunches of grass tennis courts that border the university. When it was finished in 1926, it was considered the most attractive of the science buildings in Oxford and the model of modernity in a biological research facility.

The Dunn School hardly resembled a lab of today, both in its intimacy and in its architectural detail. Immediately inside the front door is a curved oak staircase that empties into wide hallways that stretch twenty yards in either direction. One end of the building has a lecture theater with raked seats, and rooms for teaching. The other end houses the labs, in which at the time five or six scientists could comfortably work. In Dreyer's era, Oxford professors were intended to be scholars rather than administrators, and their own working accommodations were designed as a place of experiment and study rather than as an academic office. At the end of the hall on the third of three floors is the professor's suite. For its first forty years of use, the light-oak-paneled, bookshelf-lined study with a pull-down bed hidden in one of the walls was more capacious than many apartments. It connected to a large laboratory, a spacious bathroom with an eight-foot tub adorned with huge brass taps, and a sink of matching scale.

The Dunn School owed its existence to Dreyer, a Dane who was born in Shanghai, educated in Copenhagen, and studied for a period at Oxford. In 1905, he was working on diphtheria at the State Serum Institute in Copenhagen when he returned to Oxford to deliver a paper to the British Medical Association. The paper was so well received that two years later when the Chair of Pathology was established, he was elected the university's first Professor of Pathology. An immunologist, Dreyer's dedicated interest was the study of what is called the agglutination of bacteria—the reaction of particles suspended in a liquid that collect into clumps as a response to certain antibodies or sera. Antibodies are found in blood serum (which is what's left of blood after the cells are removed), and they are an important diagnostic tool for identifying the presence of invading bacteria.

Dreyer spent his first years at Oxford standardizing his methods so that the agglutinating power of a serum could be numerically quantified in units of any size, and thus could be accurately compared to other samples. His understanding of the importance of having samples of known purity later led him to establish the Standards Laboratory, which kept up-to-date pure cultures of many infecting bacteria. Scientists around the country used these so-called standard cultures of bacterial suspensions and agglutinating sera in experiments and to identify antibodies in blood samples from patients. The Standards Laboratory was so valuable that, although it remained within the School of Pathology, it became a national bank funded by the Medical Research Council, which paid rent to the Dunn School to house it.

Professors of the time were princes if not kings, and regally treated. Dreyer was imperious, and he decreed that only he and select visitors could use the front entrance to the Dunn School and the elevator.

Dreyer's success in establishing the School of Pathology was counterbalanced by the kind of humiliation that figures in every scientist's nightmares. In 1922, reports were released without his knowledge about his work on a vaccine against tuberculosis that was effective in animals. TB was a scourge, and the possibility of containing it was sensational news. The demand for the serum for clinical trials pressed Dreyer to publish his results before he had completed all his experiments. Subsequent tests by the Medical Research Council revealed that the vaccine had no effect in humans.

The blow to Dreyer's reputation was sharp but not fatal. The blow to his morale was devastating. Dreyer's scientific energy was sapped by the debacle, and this carried over to his administration of the Dunn School. In the eight years between its opening in 1926 and his death in 1934, enrollment dropped, and many of the brightest young minds went elsewhere for their training. Toward the end of his tenure, there were gross inefficiencies; one tissue section sample for study was inaccurately labeled, another was cut from a tissue block that had deteriorated. Students drifted away. The School of Pathology, one prominent scientist said, "was beginning to show some of the features of a mausoleum."

Dreyer was only sixty-one when he suddenly died during a vacation in Denmark. His death was a shock but nonetheless prompted immediate jockeying for position in the race to replace him. Because the post was at Oxford and included use of the facilities of the Dunn School, it was one of the most prestigious medical chairs in England. The job had long been in Florey's sight. Now he worried that, at thirty-six, he might be considered too young.

The centuries-old procedure for naming a new professor at Oxford was in some ways similar to that of naming a new pope, in that little was done openly. Rather, there were hidden moves and quiet proddings, political pitfalls and powerful interests. Electoral meetings were closed; minutes were not kept. Professorships established by the university are called Statutory Chairs. Each Statutory Chair at Oxford is assigned to one of the thirty-nine colleges that compose the university, and the professor is made one of its fellows; Lincoln College is responsible for the Chair of Pathology. When a chair opens, the university appoints a board to fill it. The Head of College is made an ex officio member, and the college can add a second elector. The choice of this second Lincoln elector changed the course of medicine.

Charles Sherrington, then seventy-six and about to retire as Professor of Physiology at Oxford, was eager for his protégé to get the pathology post, and from decades of experience with Oxford politics, he knew the subtle ways to influence an election. He quietly lobbied probable electors and played upon their enthusiasm for Florey as well as their fear of what the election of someone else might mean to their own position within the university. Throughout the nearly four months leading to the election, Sherrington kept Florey apprised of his efforts. Dreyer had come to see Florey as his successor, and, had he retired at age sixty-five as planned, he would have been the second Lincoln elector and a solid vote for him. The key was to get another Florey supporter on the panel.

Well into the process, Sherrington wrote with excellent news. Lincoln College had asked Edward Mellanby to be its second elector. Mellanby had moved on from Sheffield to become the secretary of the Medical Research Council and now was one of the two or three most powerful men in British medicine. As gatekeeper of medical research funding, he knew all the important work being done by the ablest scientists in Britain. Mellanby, fourteen years older than Florey, had seen him at work when both were at Sheffield. Florey was vigorous. He rolled up his sleeves and immersed himself in his work, and he performed experiments every day, all of which impressed Mellanby. Florey represented the future to Mellanby, and the selection of Mellanby as the second Lincoln elector was exactly what Sherrington had worked toward.

Sherrington also reported that his place on the electoral board had been taken by the Regius Professor of Medicine, the gloriously named Sir Farquhar Buzzard, "with whom I have been able to get two longish talks about the matter of choice for the Chair. A name *he* mentioned to me with some approval as a candidate was [Matthew] Stewart of Leeds." Buzzard was a leader in the patient-as-a-person movement that evolved after 1900. His philosophy was, "The most important difference between a good and indifferent clinician lies in the amount of attention paid to the story of the patient." He seems initially to have supported Stewart.

The Electoral Board met at Lincoln College on January 22, 1935. Every candidate's file was packed with glowing letters of recommendation. The seven distinguished scientists who wrote on behalf of Florey stressed his originality as a researcher, his ability to interest innovative collaborators, his being at the forefront of pathology, and his administrative skills. Sherrington, his most powerful nominator, concluded, "In his own special line he has, in my judgment, done things of more promise than any which preceded them for years . . . his character and attainments well fit him to fulfil with distinction and success the responsibilities of the Chair in Oxford."

Six electors were present and they discussed each candidate. Mellanby, the seventh, was not; his train from London had been beset by mechanical problems, turning an hour's journey into three. The final choice for the chair came down to Stewart of Leeds, a solid, stolid, decent man of the medical establishment whose chief qualification was an encyclopedic knowledge of morbid anatomy, and Florey, who was not at all a conventional pathologist. Stewart analyzed final results. Florey started experiments, and he was a physiologist as well as a pathologist blazing new trails. The vote was taken with Mellanby still absent. Stewart was selected.

Then just before the meeting adjourned, Mellanby arrived. Most people might feel guilty by so late an arrival. Not Mellanby, whose attitude was that he arrived in the nick of time, fortunate still to be able to save the electors from themselves. He was emphatic that Stewart was the wrong choice. Mellanby had a persuasive manner that would grow more strident in the years ahead, and he convinced the electors to reconsider their decision. Besides, money talks, and Mellanby was the money.

There is no record of the particulars of the meeting, but one of the electors later told Henry Harris, the Professor of Pathology at Oxford from 1963 to 1992, that Mellanby's argument on behalf of Florey was simple and direct. "He told them, 'If you want MRC support, I'm not going to give it to someone who looks down a microscope all the time.' " Mellanby didn't support projects, he supported people. He was an experimenter, and he wanted an experimenter in this beautiful place.

Matthew Stewart was selected because they couldn't settle on one person. But if there was someone the MRC wanted to give money to, well, that was different." Unlike elections at the University of Cambridge, where electors wait twenty-four hours to make their decisions final, decisions at Oxford are immediately set. So a few hours later the university registrar wrote to Florey, "I have the pleasure to inform you that at a meeting of the electors held here today, you were appointed Professor of Pathology, as from 1 May 1935."

Among those working in the Dunn School whom Florey inherited when he assumed his professorship was Arthur Duncan Gardner. The patrician Gardner is a perfect example of the kind of man whom, for the most part, English science had drawn into its fold for several hundred years, and whose general qualities did not change until after World War II.

Gardner, born in 1884, attended the English boarding school Rugby, where young men of breeding were trained in the Classics. "Classics were generally thought of as the only proper education of a gentleman," he wrote in his memoirs, and added, "It didn't teach you to *do* anything. Your role in life would be to make others *do* things."

He excelled at the standard curriculum of German, French, Latin, and Greek, and he left school feeling "conceited and complacent, convinced that the only really satisfactory people in the world were the English upper- and upper-middle classes, and that any deviation from their standard of speech and manners was evidence of deplorable inbreeding." He went on to study law and then bacteriology at University College, Oxford, and in 1915 was brought to the Dunn School by Dreyer, who warmed to him and then, inevitably, it seems, because of his exacting nature, later cooled; at one point, however, Dreyer considered the young man his worthy successor. In time, Gardner became the director of the Standards Laboratory and maintained the hope that one day he might still be elected. He was "disappointed" by the choice of Florey but acknowledged Florey was the more suitable choice. It was Gardner who first noticed and warned of the extreme speed with which some organisms became resistant to penicillin.

Gardner's memoir *Some Recollections* recounts the mood surrounding the change in professors:

Florey arrived and started to "clean up" the department by getting rid of all of "Dreyer's rubbish," which, according to a great friend of his in the physiology department, included the Standards Laboratory and me. There came an unpleasantly critical moment when Florey told me that he had decided to have the Standards removed to London and that he was uncertain whether to give me the option of staying in the Department to teach and research in bacteriology. To make up his mind he requested a full account of my more recent researches. I had no alternative but to provide the account, and I was much relieved when, after studying it, he invited me to stay on and take charge of the Bacteriological section, in which he did not claim to be an expert.

The opposing characteristics of Gardner and Florey could not have been starker. Gardner had the polished urbanity of the English upper middle class; Florey, the outspoken roughness of the no-nonsense Australians. As Henry Harris puts it, "Florey had a rather abrasive personality. He wouldn't call a spade a spade but he'd call it a bloody shovel. More conventional people drifted away." For all Gardner's traditional ways, he was not among those who drifted away, though he had mixed feelings about Florey: "He did not much like me, nor I him; I admired and rather envied his rich scientific background—I had . . . always felt half-educated among the scientists—and perhaps he, in his turn, slightly envied my broader based, but less effective, education." Still, although Gardner found that Florey's "inner life was closed to most of his associates, including me . . . some points of his character were manifest. He twice praised me quite generously for doing things that he said he could not have done. . . . He had therefore some basic modesty and a will to be friendly—magnanimous, perhaps." Gardner saw himself as an "ally and supporter" of Florey. He also thought him to be "an experimental pathologist of great power and no little originality."

Florey revitalized the Dunn School diplomatically and in short order. There was no mass firing of "Dreyer's rubbish," although there were reassignments. He completely revamped the teaching course, which under Dreyer had become a yearly repetition of typed lectures and unimaginative laboratory work. Unfortunately, the budget for the

Dunn School's activities for everything except Florey's salary of £1,700 (about $8,500 at the time) was just over £3,400 (about $17,000), and Florey's ambitious program was always under financial stress. He cut every expense he could, including going one step further than Dreyer. To save the £25 a year it cost to run the elevator, he forbade anyone to use it.

Within weeks after returning to Oxford, Florey set out to bring in a biochemist to help in the transformation of the Dunn School. He found him at Cambridge.

4

THE TEMPERAMENTAL CONTINENTAL

Ernst Boris Chain was twenty-nine, eight years younger than Florey, when he came to Oxford in September 1935. Both were immigrants, but any similarity stopped there. Ernst's German mother, Margarete Eisner, was related to Kurt Eisner, the Social Democrat who in November 1918 organized the overthrow of the Bavarian government only to be assassinated three months later. His grandfather was a tailor in a small town in Byelorussia and a devout Jew who spent all his free time studying the Torah and Talmud. His father, Michaelovich Chaithin, immigrated to Berlin at the end of the nineteenth century, Europeanized his name to Michael Chain, and became a chemist who built a successful company that produced chemical salts like manganese, nickel, and copper sulphates. Ernst later wrote that he was tirelessly committed to study: "I was indoctrinated by both my parents with a maxim that was beyond discussion, that the only worthwhile occupation in life was the pursuit of intellectual activities and any career which was not a university career was unthinkable."

Russian and German were spoken equally in the Chain home. Music was also a common language, and at an early age Ernst displayed an impressive ability as a pianist. He particularly enjoyed playing four-handed duets, a pleasure he would pass on to his three children. (His oldest son, Benjamin, an immunologist, found that "it was great playing together when everything was going right. But he had strong views of the technical aspect and practice could be a hazardous occupation; there would be shouting, screaming, tears. Sometimes our mother had to break it up.")

Ernst was thirteen when his father died. Within three years Germany's rampant inflation had nearly wiped out his father's estate and Chain's mother and sister, Hedwig, were forced to turn the comfortable family home into a guesthouse to make ends meet; they were able to keep their furniture only because it was required for the house to bring in money to keep creditors at bay. In 1923, Anna Sacharina, his widowed cousin from St. Petersburg, came to live with them. Twenty years his senior and childless, she would become his champion, adviser, companion, and caretaker for much of his life.

Though the circumstances of the Chain household were reduced, the pursuit of intellectual activity continued unabated. Ernst had a tutor for mathematics, dabbled in philosophy, and was schooled at the Friedrich Wilhelm University (now Humboldt University), from which he graduated with a degree in chemistry and physiology. He was attracted to the idea of explaining biological events through the actions of chemical substances and this became his lifelong approach to biochemical research. Thus it was natural that he took a particular interest in enzymes, proteins that bring about chemical action. He joined the Chemical Department of the Pathological Institute of Berlin's prestigious Charité Hospital, and, in 1930, he received his Ph.D.

In 1928, during a brighter period of the Weimar Republic, before the ascension of Hitler, Chain became a naturalized German citizen and expected to make his career there. Just what that career would be was another question. The arts were at a high peak in Weimar Germany, and Chain was entranced. His passion for music and his ability on the piano rivaled his excellence as a scientist, and for several years he wrestled with whether to make his life in the lab or in the concert hall as a professional pianist. During his studies he performed on a number of occasions in Berlin and wrote music criticism for the *Welt am Abend*, a local evening paper whose far-left-wing views reflected his own at the time but which he came to reject in later life. He also dabbled with being an impresario and, in 1930, visited the Soviet Union to arrange an exchange of musicians for the German Society of

Friends in the USSR. The following year he traveled to Argentina in the unsuccessful hope of bringing in Russian and German musicians. By then the U.S. Depression had infected the thriving economies of Europe. Although for some years to come Chain would still harbor the notion of being a pianist, in the end he chose the paycheck of science over the gamble of music, a decision no doubt influenced by the German financial crisis and the Depression, but probably even more by Anna's often reminding him about one of her brothers-in-law, a failed conductor.

In April 1933, in what appears to have been a quick decision with little or no consultation with his family, Chain left Germany, a move in keeping with his impetuous nature. He was now fluent in French (he became fluent in five languages altogether) and had come to think of France as his "second spiritual country," yet his surprising choice for a new home was England. "I left Germany," he later wrote, "because I felt disgusted with the Nazi gang, not because I thought my life was in danger. I did not believe that the system would last more than six months at the most."

When Chain got off the train in London he had £10 to his name and a stamp in his passport that prohibited him from "paid or unpaid employment," which he briskly disregarded. An uncle unenthusiastically took him in and advised that he forget looking for scientific work and take any job he could find, even delivering newspapers. Instead, Ernst wrote to Sir Frederick Gowland Hopkins, the Nobel Prize–winning head of the Sir William Dunn School of Biochemistry at Cambridge (the Dunn trustees covered every base). The school had been founded in 1927 to support research into this relatively new field under the direction of Hopkins, the leading English biochemist. Hopkins had read Chain's doctoral thesis written in Berlin, and Chain wrote to request an interview in the hope of being allowed to work in Hopkins's lab.

He asked for help as well from the Liberal Jewish Synagogue and in May was granted a one-year stipend of £250. Before an answer came from Hopkins, Chain also sought the help of another reader of his thesis, the geneticist and biologist John Burdon Sanderson Haldane. One of the most idiosyncratic (he remained an unreconstructed

Stalinist throughout his life) as well as one of the most influential scientists of the twentieth century, Haldane is particularly noted for his studies of relationships between a number of different scientific disciplines, including genetics, evolution, mathematics, and biology. He thought Chain to be an excellent scientist, and may have liked his politics as well. In May, he helped him receive a place in London's University College Hospital Medical School Department of Chemical Pathology, headed by Dr. Charles Harington.

Chain and Harington may have been a good scientific match, but the polarities of their personalities led to a preview of the difficulties Chain would face in the years ahead. With his mustache and full head of brushed-back, long curly hair, Chain looked like a better-kempt version of Albert Einstein, which was hardly the look of the average well-trimmed English scientist. Chain's flamboyant appearance was matched by his manner. He could be quite amiable; a friend remembered that "when pleased his face was shining and he reminded one of a purring kitten." When displeased, there was shouting and throwing things. "He brought to science an artistic temperament, true inspiration and originality," Florey and Fleming biographer Gwyn Macfarlane wrote.

That temperament was evident in the laboratory. Where Harington was quiet and reserved, Chain was animated and voluble: he paced the floor with his hands in constant motion, talked out loud as he worked through a problem, and was histrionic in celebration or disappointment at an experiment's outcome. Harington spoke in the refined Oxbridge accent of the educated class; Chain's English had the dissonance of an immigrant struggling with sibilance and idiom. Where the English method of scientific inquiry favored discussion among workers at all levels, the German method was strictly hierarchical—professors spoke down to their technicians, who dared not speak up. And where German scientists were used to well-equipped labs, in part because of their comfortable working relationship with industry, English labs were notoriously underequipped. As Ernest Rutherford, the father of nuclear physics, put it, "We haven't much money so we've got to use our brains." Chain complained loudly and often about inadequate equipment and berated his technicians, and it was evident quickly that he was a misfit in Harington's lab. By the summer he again was looking for a post, and again it was Haldane who came to his rescue by going to Hopkins on his behalf. In October, Chain began work in Hopkins's lab at Cambridge.

Generally and affectionately referred to as "Hoppy," Hopkins's greatest fame and his share of the 1929 Nobel Prize for physiology or medicine came from his work on the relationship between growth and diet and his elucidation of what he called "accessory food factors"—vitamins. He was perhaps the leading advocate for the notion that chemical methods could solve many biological problems. This was revolutionary thinking when, at the beginning of the twentieth century, many scientists were still persuaded by the notion of vitalism, the belief that the laws of chemistry and physics that governed other matter did not wholly explain the processes of life.

Chain called Hopkins "one of the most considerate and kindest of human beings I ever had the good fortune to meet," and Hopkins held Chain in high regard as well. Once settled at Cambridge, Chain began to modify his behavior, although he would always have what one colleague called a "rhubarbative personality." Chain referred to himself as a "temperamental Continental."

Still, he had considerable charm and was befriended by Ashley Miles, a pathologist who later became the director of the Lister Institute at the University of London, and who with some bemusement watched Chain slowly Anglicize his ways. Chain, Miles recalled, "was very proud when he had learned not to say [his technicians] were all bloody fools but to start his complaints with a quiet 'I find ziz highly disgraceful.' "

Like Chain, Miles was an ardent pianist. He regularly invited Chain to use the piano in his home and often played duets with him. Chain's solo pieces were largely by the Russian Aleksandr Scriabin, whose tortured search for the mystery of life is evident in his compositions; Chain, whose work was all about the mystery of life, was especially drawn to his late sonatas. The sessions with Miles could be "a very noisy affair," Miles later wrote, "because at the full orchestral passages Ernst wasn't satisfied with the amount of weight in the noise we were making and he would add wordless voice parts, mostly imitating the brass, in loud obbligato. We then had an upright piano and after one Bruckner session my wife swore that it had moved four inches down the wall." Chain's departure after they finished entertained Miles almost as much as Chain's company, because "Ernst's English was not very idiomatic in those days. I well remember he used to leave us after an evening visiting by saying, 'Now, *kinder*, I have the honor to retire myself.' "

The two years Chain spent at Cambridge were gratifying professionally but unsettled personally. Apart from Miles, with whom he had a solid friendship, and Hopkins, whom he admired without reservation, there was no one in the lab of whom he ever spoke with either respect or affection. He still felt the tug of desire to be a professional musician, debated whether it made sense to move to Australia or Canada, and fell victim to what he described as "frequent attacks of fear, especially in closed rooms, tube, etc." These self-termed "melancholic depressions" were almost surely psychosomatic but nevertheless real to him. Among his recurring fears was a foreboding that he would be "poisoned in the lab" and "big financial worries, uncertainty of future."

The financial worries were real enough. After the grant from the Liberal Synagogue ended, another group awarded him £300 a year while he studied for a Cambridge Ph.D. that Hopkins said would benefit him. His work in the lab paid him an additional £200 a year, barely enough to sustain him. He lived in what one friend described as "grotty digs" and did not bother much with preparing food; an invitation to the Miles home to play duets meant the added pleasure of a good meal. His persistent uncertainty about the future not only was founded on adjusting to the life of a refugee, but no doubt was exacerbated by the increasingly perilous condition for Jews in Germany. Nor was he able to arrange permission from the British government's Home Office for his cousin Anna, who had moved to Paris and started a cosmetics business with her sister, to join him in England. His musical ability brought him a circle of acquaintances beyond the lab, but even so, he spent most of 1934 feeling "uprooted and disoriented" and would be beset by these problems for the next several years. Part of Chain's emotional difficulty during this time must have stemmed from worries about his mother and sister. At the end of 1935, he received a letter, written in German by a friend with an unidentifiable signature:

> On the way to and from Moscow I met with your mother. There is no need to tell you how difficult her life is, in fact, I don't understand at all how she manages to exist. I don't know how well off you are, and I don't need to know these details. But one way or another, she needs regular monthly (financial) help and you are the only one person who can do something for her. . . .

In spite of his malaise, Chain did original work in the study of how some snake venoms attack the central nervous system and set off a series of reactions that culminate in fatal paralysis. He took the then uncommon approach of looking at the problem as a biochemical riddle: What was it in the venom, and what was its chemical structure, that instigated the chemical changes in the nervous tissue that brought about paralysis? Instead of working directly with an animal, Chain chopped up tissue, removed the cells' structural components, and then added tiny amounts of neurotoxins to the remaining chemicals. In time, he would discover that the reason such small amounts of poison can have such drastic and even fatal effects is that one enzyme in the venom destroys another enzyme in the victim's neurosystem that is critical to the control of breathing. His innovative reduction of biology to its chemical components was precisely the approach Florey wanted in his lab.

Chain was closing in on his solution when, in May 1935, Hopkins recommended him to Florey. Florey was convinced that advancement of the science of bacteriology was dependent on equal advancement in biochemistry—"Pathology will not go very well without a very big injection of chemistry into it," he said—and he wanted a solid biochemist to work with him in Oxford. He had in mind a colleague from his Cambridge days who now was working with Hopkins, and he asked Hopkins whether he might be released from his obligations there. Hopkins felt that he needed the man for at least another two years and suggested that Florey meet Chain.

"He really has become a well-qualified biochemist," Hopkins wrote. "I have just had to read his thesis for the Ph.D. degree here (which he will certainly get) and am struck with the ability it displays. . . . I feel that if his race and foreign origin will not be unwelcome in your department, you will import an acceptable and very able colleague." Chain's being Jewish was not a problem for Hopkins, but the blatant undertone of anti-Semitism was indicative of the time. Chain's often engaging personality and his talent defused it as an issue at both Cambridge and Oxford, although no amount of charm could dissipate it altogether.

Florey was ill the day Chain arrived in Oxford, so James Kent met him at the train station and they walked the couple of miles to the Dunn School. Through a window of the neighboring Dyson Perrins Lab, Chain saw a Soxhlet apparatus, which extracts the soluble portion of a substance by steady circulation of a boiling solvent through it. Although any lab today would have them in abundance, at the time Soxhlets were both rare and expensive; there might have been three or four in total in all of Oxford's labs. Kent later wrote to Gwyn Macfarlane that Chain's eyes lit up as he exclaimed, "You have Soxhlets?" One, Kent told him. "One?" he shouted in horror. "I must have six—a dozen!"

Despite the shortage of equipment, Chain soon found Oxford agreeable, as indeed Oxford found him. Chain's musicianship combined with a sympathetic feeling for political refugees at the university made for a generally easy acceptance.

Soon Chain completed his important work on snake venom with understandable pride. "For the first time," he later wrote, "the mode of action of a natural toxin of protein could be explained in biochemical terms." This was precisely the kind of original work Florey expected. To underwrite and provide stability for Chain's work, Florey arranged for a grant from the British Empire Cancer Campaign. Florey and Chain quickly established a rapport that enabled easy collaboration in their first few years together. On most days they walked home together through the University Parks. Their discussions tended more toward work than personal matters, but even so, Florey was more forthcoming with Chain than he had permitted himself to be with other contemporaries.

Florey was deeply uncomfortable around infirmity and illness—including his wife's deafness—yet he demonstrated an uncharacteristic caring in 1936 when the fears Chain had experienced in 1934 returned in full force. "Periodic fear attacks," Chain noted. "Since January increased sudden attacks of palpitations, followed by strange languor. In laboratory from time to time sudden fear of being poisoned (strong palpitations, sudden eruptions of sweat). . . . Death of several intimate friends. Several attacks of weakness, especially in the mornings." Then came the onset of severe but undiagnosable internal pains. The suspicion arose among those treating Chain that the problem might be more mental than physical, and he was sent to a place in London described by some as a nursing facility and by others as an asylum. Florey visited him there.

It was Ashley Miles who got Chain out after a mutual European friend described his plight. He had "a nervous breakdown," Miles recalled, but he felt it was wrong for Chain to have been placed in the institution. "We had him to stay during the last stages of his convalescence and our job mostly was a matter of persuading him, largely by gentle mockery from my wife, that he wasn't on the brink of collapse after every meal."

Even after his release, some physical pains persisted. Finally Anna Sacharina insisted that he come to Paris and see her doctor. While there he was introduced to Anne Beloff, a scientist whom he would later marry and collaborate with. Of more immediate importance, Anna's doctor promptly diagnosed appendicitis and, after operating on Chain, sent him back to Oxford with the removed organ bottled as a souvenir.

In 1937, Chain was able after long negotiations with the Home Office to bring Anna to Oxford as his housekeeper. She was immediately a calming influence. He was, however, unable to be of any help to his mother and sister. Jewish emigration from Germany was by then very difficult, and it is unclear that they would have been willing to leave even if allowed. In 1942, both were sent to Theresienstadt, the supposed "model Jewish settlement" in Czechoslovakia that was really a camouflage for the exportation to extermination camps, and were killed later that year.

Forever after, Benjamin Chain says, his father "didn't like to talk about pre-war Berlin, I think because he left his mother and sister and tried too late to get them out."

5

THE MICRO MASTER

Of all the major contributors to the development of penicillin, no one is so little known as Norman George Heatley, yet no one was as indispensable. Born January 10, 1911, at Woodbridge, Suffolk, he was his parents' only surviving child. Woodbridge, on the estuary of the Deben River, is an area perfectly suited to sailing, which Heatley mastered and turned into a lifelong pleasure. His father, Thomas, was a veterinarian, and as a boy, Norman would travel with him as he made his rounds of nearby farms. Thomas's skill with animals impressed Norman, but what really caught his attention was his father's talent for mending broken china by using a small hand drill to bore tiny holes for even tinier metal pins that pegged the cup or saucer together. It was a skill Thomas was able to put to good use and profit on train trips in a time when everyone carried a basket for tea and breakage was an unavoidable annoyance. His dexterity in working on a small scale would later prove to have passed from father to son, for both Norman's manual and his mental abilities would be instrumental in solving the most difficult riddle of how to extract penicillin from its multisubstance broth without rendering it impotent. His father's constant work was in contrast to his mother Grace's main occupation, which was, according to Heatley, "being an invalid."

At age seven and a half Norman was sent as a boarder to St. Felix School near Ipswich, which, he discovered, "had been a quite good one and then became the nearest thing to *The Lord of the Flies* that I ever heard of." The following year he was mercifully enrolled at West-bourne House, a boarding school on the coast in Folkstone, into whose more peaceable environment an elderly man came each week to give a demonstration of practical science that for Norman and most of the other students was the "red-letter lesson of the week" and which set him on the path to his career.

In 1929, he entered St. John's College, Cambridge, and took his degree in natural sciences, then followed that with a year studying biochemistry. As was the case with Chain, his intelligence caught the attention of Frederick Gowland Hopkins. Hopkins's lab assistant at the time was an able technician who was also a pathological hypo-chondriac prone to bouts of peering into the mirror at his throat in the belief that he was getting cancer. These instances were generally followed by a spell in the local mental hospital. One day Hopkins called in Heatley and told him, "You know James, I'm afraid he's not well. I've seen him looking at his throat again and I feel some-how that this time he'll have to be inside for quite a long time. Would you like to be my assistant? Don't tell me now, just go away and think about it."

"I'd be proud and delighted," he answered immediately.

As it turned out, James made a quick recovery without need of hospitalization, and he remained Hopkins's faithful and excellent assistant for many years to come. At first Heatley thought this left him out of a job at the height of the Depression, but soon he was awarded a grant and was able to stay on in the Dunn School, where he wrote his doctoral thesis on "The Application of Microchemical Methods to Biological Problems." Microchemical methods, used to estimate the amount of carbon, nitrogen, and other elements in substances, were a relatively new and unpopulated field based on the work of Fritz Pregl, the 1923 Nobel laureate in chemistry for his invention of the method of microanalysis of organic substances, which is to say measuring the infinitely minute. Heatley soon became one of the few scientists in Britain capable of this precise work. His grasp of the field impressed his colleagues, one of whom was Ernst Chain, who admired "his experimental neatness in general."

In early 1936, Chain, with Florey's encouragement, undertook an investigation into the carbohydrate metabolism of cancerous tumors—how they build up and break down. This work required someone proficient in microdissection and micromanipulation, and Chain, who had arrived the previous September, recommended Heatley, who had planned on founding his own commercial chemical analytical service after his time was up at Cambridge. Florey asked him to come for an interview in Oxford. "He had read all my papers. The interview was delightful. In fact, we were talking an hour and a half. He told me what he was doing and I told him some simple thing. Then a rather elderly woman I knew told me Florey was a very good chap to work with." That seemed to seal the deal, and Heatley, then twenty-five, accepted a three-year appointment paid for by an MRC grant and set aside his commercial ambitions.

The key to science is ingenuity, but its engine is money. Florey had to spend much of his time finding the cash to support the research team he had managed to assemble without the aid of even one large benefaction: most of the grants he garnered for his staff ran no longer than a year, and some were for as short as three months. Appeals to the university and the Dunn School trustees netted him a small amount to use for temporary researchers.

One was Dr. Margaret Jennings, whose father was a baron and whose mother believed that women should be as well educated as men. She was trained at the Royal Free Hospital in London and stayed on following her qualification in 1934 to work in the lab headed by Robert Webb, a bacteriologist and Florey's friend from his Cambridge days. Her work on the structure of organ tissue and the composition of cells impressed Webb, and he recommended her to Florey as a teacher and a histologist. She joined the Dunn School staff in October, just shy of her thirty-second birthday, and worked with Florey on mucous secretion and other projects; she soon became his general assistant. Her husband, Dr. Denys Jennings, a scientist in another department at Oxford, also collaborated on one project.

Although Margaret's major work with Florey was in the lab, not the least of her gifts was the ability to write easy and elegant English.

This was of particular value to the plainspoken Florey, "whose prose style," a friend recalls, "was no more elegant than his speech"—in this he resembled Fleming—and she polished the writing of his papers. (Florey's letters, however, show a supple wit and sharp sense of humor.) Despite Margaret's initial temporary status, she would work with Florey for the rest of his career. Between 1938 and Florey's death in 1968, they published thirty papers jointly or with additional authors.

Florey's longest research project was the search for money. He had taken his post as professor of pathology at Oxford just as the university received a £2 million donation from Lord Nuffield, the former William R. Morris, founder of Morris Garages, the makers of the popular Morris Minor and MG cars. The gift, equivalent to $10 million at the time, was for the support of medical research, and Florey had good reason to believe that some of that manna would find its way to the Dunn School. Unfortunately, when all the university infighting was over, the vast bulk of the money was set aside for new buildings, equipment, and endowed professorships in clinical research—as a young man Morris dreamed of being a surgeon—and little or none was available for such preclinical disciplines as pathology and biochemistry. In years to come, Nuffield would prove a financial ally to Florey. In 1936, however, Florey was denied a Nuffield grant, and he had to turn for help elsewhere. The Rockefeller Foundation was an obvious choice; Florey and foundation representatives had kept in touch since his 1925 to 1926 fellowship.

Established by John D. Rockefeller in 1913 with, by the end of 1914, an endowment of $100 million "to promote the well-being of mankind throughout the world," the Rockefeller Foundation was a great supporter of the effort to professionalize science that had begun in England in the 1850s and gained momentum following the end of World War I. The notion that experts in a particular field are the best judges of advances in the field and the most qualified to review the work of their colleagues took nearly a century to firmly root, but for the past fifty years peer review has been the bedrock on which the astonishing achievements of science rest.

A corollary to the necessity of peer review is the notion that scientists are the best people to decide which scientific research deserves financial support. In the 1920s, Edward R. Embree, then the secretary of the Rockefeller Foundation, called people who make a living giving away other people's money "philanthropoids." The Rockefeller Foundation employed a large number of these trained scientists whose job it was to travel throughout the international scientific community seeing research firsthand. They became known as "circuit riders."

Gerald Jonas writes in *The Circuit Riders: Rockefeller Money and the Rise of Science*:

> The name refers to the early disciples of John Wesley who traveled ceaselessly on horseback to bring the word of God to out-of-the-way places. . . . It is not metaphor to talk of the religious fervor that the Rockefeller circuit riders brought to their labors. In their official duties they combined the functions of seeker and missionary [and] they often spoke as if the future of humanity hung on the outcome of a race between the civilizing light of science and the dark forces of ignorance and superstition. Animated by this belief, they played an influential role in shaping the scientific community. During the decades between the two world wars, the Rockefeller Foundation set a new standard of scientific patronage.

Florey knew that Rockefeller circuit riders came to Oxford to keep up on research being done there, but he also knew that he didn't have time to wait for a random visit to promote his work in his new post. He wrote to Paris-based Daniel P. (Pat) O'Brien, the associate director of the foundation's Division of Medical Sciences, and essentially threw himself at O'Brien's feet. He explained that he had hired "a German refugee and a biochemist [Chain], supported by the Medical Research Council" and that "another biochemist [Heatley], also supported by the Medical Research Council, is coming here to work in September" to help him develop "the chemical aspect of Pathology." Florey asked for £250 ($1,280) so they could do their work. "The difficulty I find myself in at present is that the funds of the Department are inadequate for the equipment for these people." So inadequate, in fact, that Florey was unable to buy not only such necessities as a vacuum distillation apparatus, he also, Harry M. Miller of the Rockefeller Foundation later recalled, "was unable to persuade the Oxford authorities of the importance of buying common wooden kitchen tables" to hold all the petri dishes his biochemists were filling for their experiments.

O'Brien politely turned him down because the Division of Medical Sciences had quietly moved its support to psychiatry and related disciplines, but he passed on copies of their correspondence to Wilber Tisdale, the top-ranking officer in the Paris branch of the Division of Natural Sciences. O'Brien said to Tisdale that he would have liked to help Florey and that he felt the request "should be carefully considered under any circumstances, because of Florey's importance and the significance of the development at Oxford." This recognition of Florey's appointment to the Chair of Pathology is an indication of the foundation's larger support for what Jonas calls "the progressive wing of the British scientific community," represented in part by Sherrington and Mellanby.

Two weeks later, on June 15, 1936, Tisdale visited Florey in Oxford and reported back to Paris that Florey needed "balances, micro balances, vacuum distillation apparatus, etc. to a value of about £250. The MRC does not give equipment, the Royal Society is swamped with applications, and the university is not willing to help him further. F. is an exceptionally good man and he is working on interesting problems, but they are not directly in either MS or NS programs." On June 26, Florey had his grant. By the time Heatley arrived in Oxford in September, the money was already well spent.

Once settled in, Heatley and Chain began their experiments on cancerous tumors and eventually discovered that there was no difference in the metabolism of normal skin and malignancies. In the course of their work, Heatley designed and built a microrespirometer for measuring the respiration of and the energy exchanged by tiny tissue fragments containing a minute number of cells. Heatley's device, made from odds and ends and parts of his own manufacture, is such an original piece of machinery that it is on exhibit in London in the Science Museum.

Along with many other specialists on the Dunn School staff, Heatley and Chain also were part of a joint investigation of the biochemistry of lymphocytes. Lymphocytes normally compose 25 percent of the body's white blood cells, but they increase in number as T and B cells are created to fight infections. This systematic approach of independent scientists functioning as members of an informal team, each solving his own parts of a larger puzzle, was at the time an uncommon approach in British science, but it was central to Florey's overall plan for revitalizing the Dunn School, and it was an indication of Mellanby's faith in his vision. Heatley's delicate application of micromethods deepened the understanding of the metabolism of lymphocytes. This multitalented approach was vital to the work that led to the development of penicillin and subsequent advancements.

All members of a team do not necessarily have to like one another to accomplish great things; they simply have to find ways to do their work in a way that minimizes the distractions of personality clashes. Heatley and Chain began their collaboration with high hopes and relative ease. Indeed, when Heatley came to Oxford he wrote, "I could hardly believe my good fortune and I resolved to do my best to justify it." But he and Chain were opposites in temperament, in personality, in scientific approach, and even in appearance: Heatley was well trimmed and rail-thin, Chain was hirsute and hardy; Heatley was reticent and shy, Chain was voluble and demonstrative; Heatley wrote meticulous notes, Chain took few notes; Heatley was invariably courtly, Chain could be curt; Heatley was reluctant to seek credit, Chain was quick to claim his due. Heatley had little exposure to the world outside England, though his future travels would change this; his experience and outlook were provincial, while Chain's were more international. Chain was unlike anyone Heatley had met before.

While Heatley had been brought to Oxford as Chain's assistant, a role he was grateful to assume, he soon felt that he was doing far more than a normal assistant. He also felt that "the more I did the more was expected," and he found that he rather than Chain "was perhaps better at actually *doing* research; I had a better grasp of the practical side, with reasonable experimental aptitude." Chain, whose German training specified that the senior scientist was followed with alacrity and without question, expected no less of Heatley; Heatley, brought up in a far more collegial method, chafed at Chain's expectation of unquestioned obedience. Heatley, impeccably mannered and possessed by a palpable sense of deference, cites a "trivial example" of behavior that set him on edge. Chain required a scarce enzyme for a project he was working on without Heatley's help. Heatley knew of someone who had worked with the enzyme and was asked ("almost 'ordered' ") to write and request some, which was duly and generously sent. Heatley suggested that Chain warmly thank the donor but says Chain's response was, "You can write him if you want, but he is not a very interesting or important person." Heatley was offended by Chain's recurrent "contempt for inferiors, coupled with ingratiating servility towards those in higher places or likely to be useful."

Another, not at all trivial source of Heatley's disenchantment occurred over the publication in the *Biochemistry Journal* of the details of the microrespirometer. Forty years later he wrote "with reluctance" in response to being asked to set the record straight that "it was wholly my conception and design. [Chain] explained that he could not afford not to put his name to the paper because he had to make a career in this country, a point I accepted with some resentment. It is quite clear that I myself was also striving for kudos, but I felt that a) it was deserved, and b) my future might well hang on it." According to Heatley, when the question of the order of authors' names came up, Chain argued that the journal's policy was to list them alphabetically, but most likely it was Florey who ruled that Heatley's should come first, and it does. Chain's recollection differed: "Some frictions arose regarding the publication of the authorship of papers which seemed to me quite unnecessary and indicated a certain pettiness and lack of generosity in Heatley's character."

Two bright men who at first looked as if they would combine their talents into an amiable partnership by now combined no better than oil and water. Heatley had a fierce and stubborn pride in his ability. *He* knew his contribution to every project, and if others did not have the intelligence to notice the value of his work, that was their loss. Of course in many instances it was Heatley's loss as well, because many times his inventive work critical to success went unnoticed or, as in the case of his contribution to the development of penicillin, long undervalued. Within a few months Heatley quietly had "forfeited [his] respect" for Chain. Florey, however, never hesitated to differ with Chain, who described how "the very walls of Florey's office would shudder" from the intensity of their arguments.

Regardless of these problems, Chain and Heatley continued to work together, and Chain had other collaborators on at least five separate inquiries as he looked into subjects as varied as the biochemistry of venoms and toxins and the chemistry of gastric function. This was a period of excellent work by Chain. He published seven scientific papers in two years, created a thriving biochemistry department within the Dunn School, and aimed to do even more. His personal financial situation had improved, but he still was on the lookout for subjects that would bring long-term grants, a constant concern of Florey's as well; both men were frustrated by how little research money there was available in general and to them in particular. Finding financial support for work to be done over a period of years was as challenging as the scientific work being undertaken by the Dunn School staff. In fact, by 1938, the school was overdrawn in its accounts by as much as £500, and Florey banned the purchase of any equipment and even stationery. Only the most important letters went out under the Dunn School letterhead; the rest, even Florey's, were written on ordinary typing paper embossed with a hand die.

Before Chain and Heatley completed their tumor study, Florey asked Chain to apply his energies to the study of lysozyme, a substance that had interested Florey for eight years, in part because it appears in duodenal secretions and therefore could have some effect on ulcers. Because lysozyme appeared to be an enzyme and because technically it was closely related to the work Chain had already done on snake venom, the inquiry also was of particular interest to him. Little was known about lysozyme's chemistry, and Chain was excited by the prospect of discovery. Along with an American Rhodes scholar, Leslie A. Epstein, he showed that lysozyme was in fact an enzyme, as Fleming suspected. Building on Fleming's initial work, the two isolated lysozyme and deciphered its chemical nature, an achievement that biographer Macfarlane called a "brilliant solution," and which Chain felt began a new "chapter of biomedical research . . . the chemical nature of the bacterial cell wall."

Chain and Epstein showed that the enzyme worked by dissolving a complex carbohydrate called a nitrogenous polysaccharide. Alas, as Fleming's more primitive work had shown, this dissolvable molecule is not present in any microbes that cause serious human diseases and therefore lysozyme had no effect on them. While the work explained how cell walls were destroyed, it did not lead toward the discovery of other antibacterial substances, and so, however original the work, for Florey, this was a dead end. (It was also a precursor; Florey and Chain's leadership in the resolution of the properties of a substance first noticed by Fleming would be repeated with penicillin.) Actually, this work done during 1937 and 1938 turned out to be particularly fortuitous.

Chain's approach to a problem was to read as much as he could about how similar investigations were carried out. In the age before computer searches, this meant poring over journals issue by issue, in this case looking for similar instances of enzyme activity and antibacterial action along the lines of lysozyme. This was not an unknown area to Florey, who after all was an editor of the *British Journal of Experimental Pathology* when it published Fleming's paper on penicillin in 1929, although it seems he had long forgotten about it. Of more importance, in 1930, Florey coauthored a paper on bacterial antagonism with reference to two reviews of other work on the subject, but surprisingly not to the obvious one, Fleming's paper on penicillin. Florey's friend and colleague Edward Abraham later wrote, "It is difficult to believe that [Florey and his coauthor] were unaware of the striking example of microbial antagonism which had been described by Fleming in the same journal in 1929." But apparently they were. On hearing of Chain's interest in antibacterial action, Florey told him bacterial antagonism had been an interest of his since 1929, and he suggested that Chain look at a 1928 paper by G. Papacostas and J. Gaté, *Les Associations Microbiennes*, which has a sixty-page chapter on "antibiosis" (from the Greek meaning "against life") and cites several hundred references.

"Antibiosis" was first used by Jean-Paul Vuillemin, in 1889, to describe the fight for survival between two living beings. In his paper entitled "Antibiosis and Symbiosis," he described how fungi and yeasts can destroy bacteria. Then he added: "No one considers the lion which leaps upon its prey to be a parasite nor the snake which injects venom into the wound of its victim before eating it. Here there is nothing equivocal; one creature destroys the life of another to preserve its

THE MICRO MASTER | 79

own. . . . The one is in complete opposition to the life of the other. The conception is so simple that no one has ever thought of giving it a name."

Chain later wrote that he collected "about 200 references on growth inhibitions caused by the action of bacteria, streptomycetes, fungi and yeast on one another," and carefully read each. He learned how little was known. "It was evident that in many cases the growth inhibition was caused by specific metabolites produced by various micro-organisms. However, next to nothing was known about the chemical or biological nature of the inhibitory substances, and it seemed an interesting and rewarding field of exploration."

Then one day early in 1938, he came upon Fleming's paper on penicillin in one of the many bound volumes of the *British Journal of Experimental Pathology,* a find he described as "sheer luck." It was not so much luck that a biochemist would be reading a journal of pathology—although most biochemists wouldn't naturally turn to a pathology journal, Chain, after all, was working in a school of pathology—and he probably had already found Fleming's two papers on lysozyme as well as the two by Florey in other volumes. It was Fleming's name and the third word in the paper's title ("On the Antibacterial Action of Cultures of a Penicillium with Special Reference to Their Use in the Isolation of B. Influenzae") that caught his eye. When he read Fleming's presumption that penicillin destroyed bacteria by lysis—that is, it dissolves bacteria rather than producing a substance that kills them—Chain thought it possible that penicillin was similar to lysozyme in how it acted and therefore worthy of more study.

Chain was "immediately interested," as he later explained.

The reason was that, according to Fleming's description, the mould had strong bacteriolytic properties against the staphylococcus. . . . I thought Fleming had discovered a sort of mould lysozyme, which, in contrast to egg white lysozyme, acted on a wide range of gram-positive pathogenic bacteria. I further thought that in all probability the cell wall of all these pathogenic bacteria whose growth was inhibited by penicillin contained a common substance on which this supposed enzyme acted

... it would, of course, be necessary to purify the supposed enzyme, but I did not foresee any undue difficulties. . . .

His further search of the literature led him to Raistrick's 1932 paper and to the probable conclusion that penicillin would turn out to be an enzyme. Chain later wrote that he decided to look into the substance "because it would have shown us something about the structure of the cell of pathogenic bacteria and we should have isolated a constituent of obviously vital importance from the bacterial cell which was common to a large number of pathogens."

By remarkable coincidence, to find a sample of *Penicillium notatum* to work with he had to go no farther than across the corridor to the lab of Margaret Campbell-Renton, who had been Georges Dreyer's assistant. Chain remembered that soon after he came to the Dunn School, he had seen her in the hallway carrying a tray of petri dishes with a mold culture, and so he wandered over and asked her if she knew of *Penicillium notatum*. She not only knew about it, she had a culture that had been growing at the Dunn School for years. It was probably Dreyer who had asked for the culture because he thought that the active ingredient in penicillin might be a bacteriophage, a virus that infects and kills bacteria. When he found it wasn't, he abandoned his inquiry. Over the next decade, Campbell-Renton kept the mold growing along with the others in the school's collection, using some of the penicillin in the bacteriology lab as a sort of biological hit man to kill unwanted bacteria from cultures of *Bacillus influenza,* which was not sensitive to it.

Chain took some penicillin mold back to his lab and with Epstein performed a few experiments with it to try to understand a bit about its nature. Their inability to reproduce Fleming's results dispelled his notion that penicillin was a sort of lysozyme. But the very difficulties of penicillin—its makeup, its instability, the problems with extracting it—made Chain believe that it was quite singular and therefore of particular scientific interest. He was not put off by the published failures of Fleming and of Raistrick, whom he felt could not have been much of a chemist if he couldn't get penicillin into a stable form. Chain felt certain that penicillin was not as labile as they had assumed because, he told Florey, any chemical that will keep in an ice chest for months "is subject to chemical manipulation."

The details of how Florey and Chain came to undertake the studies that led to the development of penicillin are so sketchily documented that they are impossible to reconstruct in full. This would be of no particular consequence had not their amicable relationship disintegrated during the 1940s. In the years to come, Chain would feel that his contribution was not properly credited; by the late 1940s, he and Florey communicated only in writing.

Chain would later argue that on a number of occasions over a period of many months, he brought penicillin to Florey and that it was not until the fall of 1939 that Florey turned his energy to it. "Remember, no one is alive who was present at the talks which took place between Florey and myself during 1938 and 1939," he wrote to Gwyn Macfarlane in 1978, "so no one apart from myself can possibly know what was said in these talks. I can assure you that the word penicillin was never mentioned by Florey to me until I told him that I had started work on it."

That may be so, but David Masters, whose 1946 book, *Miracle Drug: The Inner History of Penicillin*, drew heavily on interviews with Florey and Chain, wrote that it was in 1938 that

Professor Florey concluded that the anti-bacterial substances offered almost a virgin field for pure research, so he discussed the matter in all its aspects with Dr. Chain. The idea appealed to both men. . . . Professor Florey could deal with the biological problems, while Dr. Chain could work out the chemical problems. . . . But much had to be done before it could be started, and Dr. Chain resumed his search of the literature until his notes were complete.

At length Dr. Chain and Dr. Florey sat down together to survey the field and . . . planned [researches that] were purely academic, of interest to science alone. . . . Their aim was . . . to conduct researches into every [bacterial antagonist] known, but eventually they narrowed the field to three subjects, *Bacillus pyocyaneus* [now *Pseudomonas pyocyanea*], *Penicillium notatum*, and *Subtilis-mesentericus*.

Like lysozyme, all three substances had bacteriolytic action. But which bacterium should they study first? Penicillin's odd chemistry appealed to Chain; that it was potent against staphylococcus appealed to Florey. As they walked home one evening, they decided this was the place to start. There was no clap of thunder, no mental lightbulb that turned on; there was no way to know they had stepped onto an historic path.

Florey needed continuing research money, and he was determined to get it, even if it meant gambling on an investigative long shot. Four years of MRC support for the investigation of lysozyme had, Florey admitted, "produced nothing." Penicillin could just as well lead to another dead end, but something that could lead to a big result had to be undertaken.

"There is no question, we will have to go for penicillin," Florey told his friend R. Douglas Wright, an Australian physiologist whom he had brought to Oxford on a fellowship. "My worry is that I've got the bacteriologists and the biologists, and I've got my team together. If the money doesn't come along, I might not be able to hold them together and it would all be finished."

About half of the school's operating income came from the university, another quarter came from the Dunn Endowment Fund, and the remainder was from student fees and small grants that Florey said he "found by shaking a hat in all possible directions," the main direction being toward the MRC. Despite periods of mutual irritation, Mellanby wanted to provide Florey with as much support as he could. Wright, who worked with Florey on mucous secretion in 1937, later wrote to Macfarlane that at the Physiological Congress in Zurich in mid-1938, Mellanby told him "that he was having trouble keeping funds available for Florey's antibacterial materials programme, and was telling Florey that he must make one full-blooded throw . . . in late November 1938, Florey told me of his plan to go all out for penicillin."

The MRC was suffering from the same lack of funds as the scientists in Oxford and elsewhere. Poverty can strain even the closest relationships. Where mutual sympathy might have been the logical consolation for Florey and Mellanby, instead there were periods of mutual testiness. Florey complained that he had "the utmost difficulty in finding money for even relatively small essentials in my work." Mellanby in turn complained to Daniel O'Brien of the Rockefeller Foundation that instead of concentrating on meaningful research, his golden boy was playing at "Oxford medical politics," and that it was time to "prove himself." Six weeks later, Mellanby told Wilber Tisdale that Florey "was having a very difficult time attempting to reorganize and rearrange his laboratory . . . and this was at the moment complicated by too many irons in the fire at the same time."

Mellanby had his own political problems. The MRC was funded by Parliament on a five-year cycle; the last disbursement, in 1934, had been for £1 million. Now, however, more was being allocated in grants than was projected in the budget, and Mellanby had to scramble to cover his expenses; he even transferred £10,000 out of a £30,000 special fund he had set aside for nutritional studies, his own scientific specialty. Mellanby hoped that the Rockefeller Foundation would be his knight in sterling armor.

Florey was also at the Zurich congress in 1938, along with the Rockefeller Foundation's Tisdale. A part of each congress was set aside for eulogies of prominent physiologists who had died since the last meeting. Among those honored this time was John D. Rockefeller Sr., who had died in May 1937. Although Rockefeller was not a scientist, Tisdale noted the congress's appreciation that through his foundation Rockefeller "had undoubtedly done more for physiology than any other one man."

Florey needed no reminder of the importance of Rockefeller's benevolence, and he took advantage of the occasion to inquire whether the foundation could help him yet again. The MRC grants that supported valuable members of his team would end in about six months, he faced a life-or-death situation, and he wondered whether the foundation would be able to give him a three-year grant of £600 to £700 per year to "keep this team in existence."

This time, Tisdale could offer no encouragement. The circuit riders had spent much of their money aiding scientists and scholars from Germany and other countries faced with tyranny, and there was nothing left for small discretionary grants. If Florey wanted to be considered for Rockefeller support, he would have to submit a proposal for a more ambitious line of research. The best long-term project Florey had at hand was his and Chain's investigation of microbial antagonism. As Florey said in an informal talk in 1944 to a group of Yale medical students, "The lysozyme question was coming to an end. Chain and I in endeavoring to extract money from the Rockefeller Foundation produced a plan for a study of antibacterial substances, the antibiotics."

With Florey's injunction against the purchase of any new supplies still fresh in his mind, Chain later said that, under the circumstances, their decision put them in "an almost impossible situation in which to start planning a new branch of work."

6

"WITHOUT HEATLEY,
NO PENICILLIN"

By the end of 1938, Winston Churchill's 1935 warning to Parliament of "Germany arming at breakneck speed, England lost in a pacifist dream, France corrupt and torn by dissension, America remote and indifferent" was no longer a rhetorical flourish but a dangerous fact. It was now evident that sooner rather than later, Britain would be at war, regardless of Prime Minister Neville Chamberlain's deluded assurance that September of "peace for our time." (The phrase is a hopeful borrowing from a versicle in the Anglican service of Evensong: "Give peace in our time, O Lord. / Because there is none other that fighteth for us, but only thou, O God.")

From the largest cities to the smallest villages, citizens prepared their civil defense. Air-raid shelters were designated, blackout curtains for homes sewn; gas masks were distributed, fire wardens named. At the Dunn School, Heatley noted in his diary, "several people in the lab . . . began digging trenches near the bicycle sheds" on the boundary of the school grounds. "This went on for three days." The usual pictures of film stars and athletes on the trading cards included in at least one company's packages of cigarettes were replaced with a series of forty-eight "Air-Raid Precautions" drawings with such titles as "Rendering your refuge room gas-proof" and "Removal of incendiary bomb with scoop and hoe." Plans were made to evacuate hundreds of thousands of people from the large cities, presumed to be most vulnerable to attack, and distribute them in rural areas. Major hospitals were organized into the Emergency Medical Service; those closest to a city's center were reserved for expected casualties from air raids and other ravages of war. The Radcliffe Infirmary, Oxford's hospital, was designated the Emergency Medical Service Hospital for the Oxford area. In the event of war, the Radcliffe also was designated as a place of refuge for patients from London medical school hospitals and a place for their students to continue their studies.

It was against this backdrop that in January 1939, Florey made his first formal mention of penicillin in a grant request to the MRC for Chain and Epstein to continue "work on lytic substances . . . as well as the nature of the antibacterial substance in 'penicillin' and 'actinomycetin,' " but it would be another eight months before a detailed grant request was made.

Florey, concerned about keeping his team together in the event of war, received unexpected help from the War Office. It offered to pay the department if Florey would put in one-third of his time, if needed, as a consultant on poison gas research. With the assistance of the War Office and the MRC, Florey devised a plan with the Ministry of Health to make his pathologists a research group with a specialty in blood transfusion. A transfusion service was set up with Chain as the head and Dr. Gordon Sanders of the Dunn School staff as Area Transfusion Officer. Insultingly, Chain, even though he had taken an appropriate Red Cross First Aid course, was later forbidden to work on patients with the transfusion team he headed because he was an alien. Sanders, whose ingenuity in the lab almost equaled Heatley's, was originally to be posted at Reading, twenty-five miles away, but Florey did not want to lose his services in the lab and successfully appealed the decision, keeping him and his war post in Oxford. Ethel Florey, able to have a meaningful job at last, headed the teams of doctors from the local medical staffs who would gather blood from donors.

"She was very much in charge," wrote Gwyn Macfarlane, one of the doctors under her command. "Good-looking and invariably well dressed, she impressed her teams of young Radcliffe doctors with her undoubted charm tempered with a steely determination that made for efficiency through trepidation. She wore a double tortoise-shell ear trumpet that curved beneath her hair, and there was a general agreement that her hearing was selective, in the sense that, in the event of an argument, it was her opponent's most telling points that seemed inaudible. . . . Probably for the first time since her marriage she was able to take an active part in affairs beyond her purely domestic world."

These preparations for war, which continued through the first nine months of 1939 and naturally took a considerable amount of Florey's time, are at least a partial explanation of why, considering he had already made up his mind about pursuing antibiotics, it was many months before the grant applications were completed. In addition, this was a particularly robust period of research into other subjects. In 1938 and 1939, Florey, in conjunction with various colleagues, published four papers on mucous secretion in guinea pigs, cats, and pigs; two on observations of transparent tissue in the rabbit's ear chamber; one on lysozyme in egg white and cat and human saliva; and another on the relation of gastric secretion to red blood cells. Plus, he made a film on microcirculation.

Then there was the problem of growing enough penicillin to start a thorough investigation. This required expertise Chain did not have in working with mold as well as in the art of brewing, because the making of penicillin is a process of fermentation. For the first few months, it took ten days or more to produce active penicillin, and at least another fifteen hours to perform the imprecise bacteriological tests to determine how active the material was. Chain was in the difficult position of trying to measure the vitality of something he was able to make in only small amounts: in order to gain a higher yield, he had to understand its biochemical makeup; yet to discern the biochemical makeup, he needed a larger supply of penicillin. His only recourse was to make the most educated guess of how to proceed and trust this would lead him somewhere useful. As each of these experiments took two or three weeks to complete, it was very slow going. (Florey and the others at Oxford used the term *penicillin* to name the actual antibiotic substance derived from the mold juice; Fleming called the mold juice itself penicillin. Florey often said later that had he and his group applied a new name to the active material, it would have avoided much confusion and conflict over credit for the drug.)

Florey kept abreast of Chain's work during this period, but there were many other demands on his time, not least his constant scramble for research money. An application to a committee of the Nuffield Medical Benefaction for a £200 yearly grant to pay Margaret Jennings's salary to collaborate with him on studies of gut function was, Florey complained to Mellanby on June 11, "turned down in contemptuous terms." One of the committee members was Sir Farquhar Buzzard, who likely voted against Florey's election as Professor of Pathology in 1935.

"You told me the other day, when you came to the department, that you had to take off your shirt to meet requests—I hope you have another one," Florey continued. "The difficulties of trying to keep work going here are more than I am prepared to go on shouldering as it seems to me that I have acquired a reputation of being some sort of academic highway robber because I have to make such frequent applications for grants from all sorts of places." Heaped on this aggravation was the university's plan to reduce his operating grant because a new heating plant was expected to lower costs. "I have struggled to keep the place warm on money I ought to have devoted to research. . . . You may gather that I am fed up."

Mellanby was sympathetic and philosophical in his response, reminding Florey that he had always intellectually and financially supported "your attempts to get the Pathology Department at Oxford into an active state, and that this sympathy has been shown in a number of cases in a practical way. I don't think you ought to be disturbed, your efforts have had great success, but I am quite sure that if you want to keep that place going you will always have some kind of struggle, so that you had better resign yourself to it."

However taxing were Florey's troubles, they paled in light of what was happening in Europe. On March 15, Hitler invaded Czechoslovakia; at the end of March, he annexed Austria. In early April, Benito Mussolini ordered the Italian army to invade Albania. On May 22, the Nazis signed the "Pact of Steel" with Italy. On August 23, the Nazis and the Soviet Union signed a nonaggression pact; on August 25, Britain and Poland signed a Mutual Assistance Treaty.

Life at the Dunn School alternated between research and readiness. There was great fear of the powerful incendiary bombs dropped by the Luftwaffe, and in the summer of 1939 every able-bodied man at the school was called on to dig an air-raid shelter in a vegetable patch behind the building. Five-year-old Charles Florey was particularly active in the supervision of the work.

Also that summer, a key member of the Dunn School team prepared to leave. Heatley, whose three-year grant was about to expire, was awarded a Rockefeller Traveling grant to study in Copenhagen with the esteemed biochemist Dr. Kaj Ulrik Linderstrøm-Lang. He planned to go on September 12. Then on September 1, the Nazis invaded Poland, and, on September 3, Britain, France, Australia, and New Zealand declared war against Germany. Suddenly, travel made no sense.

Few spoiled plans have come to greater good. Had Heatley departed as scheduled, without doubt the work on penicillin would have suffered and quite possibly not succeeded at all. In apportioning the credit for penicillin's development, Henry Harris links the four principal scientists: "Without Fleming, no Chain or Florey; without Chain, no Florey; without Florey, no Heatley; without Heatley, no penicillin."

With Heatley staying at Oxford, his dexterity with micromethods could be put to good use. Florey asked him if he would be willing to work with Chain on penicillin, a substance Heatley had known about since the early 1930s when it was mentioned in a lecture at Cambridge and he had looked up Fleming's paper. Heatley said that although the work sounded very interesting, his lack of regard for Chain would make it impossible for him to continue as his assistant. Florey then suggested that Heatley become *his* personal assistant and report to him but that he continue to work with Chain, an arrangement that Heatley immediately accepted. Chain later wrote that he had not known about either Heatley's unwillingness to work with him or his new role as Florey's assistant until more than thirty years later, and that as a result "I understand now many actions of Heatley which were inexplicable to me at the time."

Florey arranged to have Heatley's Rockefeller grant paid to the MRC, which in turn passed it on to Oxford as Heatley's salary. In his letter to the foundation Florey wrote, "It is very unfortunate for Heatley that he cannot carry on his programme as he has been left through no fault of his own without any source of income for the past six weeks, which he finds somewhat difficult."

This change in working conditions was a huge relief for Heatley, who immediately found that "daily work was much pleasanter and less time wasted. Florey was in many ways the antithesis of [Chain]. He listened carefully to the views of the least experienced of his research staff, such as myself, and one could have a thoughtful and productive two-way talk with him. On occasion this could be intensely stimulating. One quickly learned that his advice was perceptive and often unexpectedly valuable, being presented in some modest form such as 'You might consider . . . ,' or 'I doubt if you are right there, but why not try it. . . .' He was generous in giving maximum credit to his colleagues, and if he gave an undertaking this could be utterly relied on. . . . I had plenty of work and plenty of ideas, and, under Florey, had the freedom, encouragement and when needed, the advice, to pursue them."

The two men would work together for over thirty years, but Heatley would always feel that Florey was greatly superior to him in academic rank and accomplishment and maintained a formal relationship; he always referred to Florey as "the Professor." For all his ease in working with Florey, Heatley felt he was "not the kind of person you said to, 'Let's go have a cup of tea.' " Even on the few occasions one was in the other's home—it was an easy walk between them—Heatley was always uncomfortable and at a loss for conversation, so great was his esteem.

On September 6, 1939—three days after Britain's entry into the war—Florey made his first detailed appeal for support of work on penicillin.

"I enclose some proposals which I think might be profitably carried out by Chain and myself," he wrote to Mellanby. There was "no really effective substance against bacteria *in vivo*"—a living being—and he "had long had the feeling that something might be done along these lines," adding: "There is little doubt that Chain has a great flair for dealing with enzyme proteins and the proposals now made have a very practical bearing at the moment."

He laid out the work done on lysozyme and while admitting that "its action is almost entirely confined to non-pathogenic organisms," he pointed out that there were accounts in the scientific literature of other, more powerful antibacterial substances, among them strains of penicillium, actinomyces—bacteria found in mucus—and certain soil bacteria. He cited Fleming's discoveries of penicillin's effectiveness against staphylococci and other bacteria and added with a buoyancy he would soon regret that "penicillin can easily be prepared in large amounts and is non-toxic to animals, even in large doses. Hitherto the work on penicillin has been carried out with very crude preparations and no attempt has been made to purify it. In our opinion the purification of penicillin can be carried out easily and rapidly.

"In view of the possible great importance of the above mentioned bactericidal agents it is proposed to prepare these substances in a purified form suitable for intravenous injections and to study their antiseptic action *in vivo*," which would test penicillin's effectiveness in a living body rather than simply in a petri dish.

This request is significant not just because of what it led to but because it is so uncharacteristic of Florey's usual grant-writing style. Gwyn Macfarlane, who knew Florey, Chain, and Heatley, was convinced that the "airy optimism" regarding the easy growth and purification "must have been inspired by Chain," and that the reference to nontoxicity in animals, which could have been based only on Fleming's injection of one mouse and one rabbit, leads to the supposition that "Chain's enthusiasm overcame Florey's scientific caution."

It is also significant that Florey's request raised the possibility that there was something of therapeutic value to humans in penicillin. Both Chain and Florey would later categorically say that penicillin's worth as a possible drug was not what caught their interest; rather, they only were drawn to it from scientific interest. "People sometimes think that I and the others worked on penicillin because we were interested in suffering humanity. I don't think it ever crossed our minds," Florey said many years later.

That may have been true when they first turned to it after lysozyme, but with the outbreak of war and with the clear understanding that they had to aim high if they wanted long-term funding, Florey pulled out all the stops, and on at least one occasion acknowledged that he was aware there might be medical use for penicillin as well: "It's always in the background of people working in medical subjects that it might be of use in medicine, but that's not the mainspring of why they do their researches." Also, behind Florey's rather gruff public face there was a sincere vulnerability. The letters to Ethel when she was still in Australia show him to be, a friend wrote, "sensitive, lonely, unsure of himself, and deeply concerned for human troubles—a picture of himself very different from the one he presented to the world." Referring to untreatable infections, he wrote in 1923 of "the appalling thing of seeing young people maimed or wiped out while one can do nothing." Henry Harris points out that "a glance at his publications shows that nothing he did was far removed from some major human disease."

For all its high ambition, the initial request to the MRC was for only £100, for "media for growing organisms, and special chemicals and apparatus," and for Mellanby's validation of the enterprise in general. Two days later, Mellanby responded: "You can assume that we will give you £25 for expenses for this work and will remember your application for £100 for expenses when the time comes for a proper decision."

This minuscule largesse was symptomatic of the MRC's own financial problems but even so, £25—something around $100—to begin a whole new scientific undertaking is rather breathtaking. And Mellanby actually liked the proposal: "It seems to me," he added, "that the line of work you are suggesting will be interesting and may prove of practical importance."

In October, Florey suggested to Chain that he make his own application to the MRC for support, the first time he would do so on his own. It was a mark of his rising stature. In short order he received the promise of £300 yearly until 1943, and expenses of £250 per year for 1939 and 1940 for work on "naturally occurring antibacterial substances." While this provided Chain with a living wage, it did not resolve the larger problem of how to properly fund research at the Dunn School instead of having to rely on what he called "those little bits and pieces of £50 and £100 . . . which did not lead us anywhere." He urged Florey to apply to the Rockefeller Foundation for a substantial enough grant to let them do real work. The approach would be two-pronged: Chain would concern himself with isolating antimicrobial substances, while Florey would look into their biological and pharmaceutical properties.

Their timing could not have been better. On November 1, the Rockefeller Foundation's Paris-based circuit rider Harry Miller, himself a bacteriologist, came to Oxford to see the highly regarded chemist Robert Robinson at the Dyson Perrins Laboratory and then walked the couple of hundred yards down South Parks Road to drop in for a visit with Florey at the Dunn School, whose outside walls now were protected by stacks of sandbags and whose labs were filled with evacuees from various London institutions. These refugees far outnumbered Florey's staff. Among them were scientists from the Emergency Public Health Laboratory Service, who had "invaded" (to use Heatley's word) the Dunn School in October and taken over almost the whole of the first floor and a large part of the basement. After they departed in 1946, Florey sent the MRC photos of the deplorably dirty condition they had allowed their quarters to fall into.

Other invasions were more worrisome. Nazi bombs had already fallen on Edinburgh and further air raids were inevitable. Virtually everyone Miller saw carried a gas mask.

Florey told Miller that he was about to ask the foundation to provide about £1,500 a year for three years to fund an investigation of "naturally produced bacteriological inhibitors . . . [that] stop in a striking way the growth of staphylococci." Miller "raised his eyebrows meaningfully," Florey later said, and intimated that Florey would stand a much better chance of being funded if he cast his application as a biochemical rather than a medical investigation because there was an overabundance of requests for the latter. Going through the foundation's Natural Sciences Division instead of its Division of Medical Sciences also bypassed Mellanby and the MRC in the negotiation of the grant request, a detour that would annoy Mellanby when he learned about it a year later.

Miller reported to Warren Weaver, head of the Natural Sciences Division, in New York that Florey needed a multiyear commitment because "In spite of the uncertainties of the war situation he [Florey] felt that the work could go on unless Oxford were almost totally destroyed by bombing; and felt that he would have to have assurances over a three-year period as it would be practically impossible to secure the necessary trained personnel on a year to year basis." Miller thought this entirely reasonable: "F. practically is the only experimental pathologist of any real distinction in the British Isles. [He] is a distinguished young investigator who has the full confidence of Mellanby and [I feel] that his request if and when received should be given serious study."

Gerald Jonas, an adept reader between the lines of intra–Rockefeller Foundation correspondence, notes: "RF officers customarily muted their enthusiasm in official correspondence. But from the special attention Miller gave this report, Warren Weaver must have guessed [that Miller] was more than a little excited about what he called 'this bacteriological inhibitor business.' "

War complicated the logistics of correspondence. Following standard practice, Miller sent one copy of every important memo to New York via the Pan American Airways Clipper that flew from Lisbon (total travel time even with the largest portion by air was about a week) and another via sea mail, so that if one carrier was shot down or sunk, the mail would still get through. But this time Miller also cabled a lengthy—and therefore expensive—report to New York that, though it centered on the work of other British scientists more eminent than Florey, gave prominence to his proposal.

One reason for Miller's deluge of information was that the Rockefeller board was about to meet. With the United States still neutral, the question of whether the foundation would follow a rising tide of isolationist sentiment in the States and reduce its presence in Europe was still to be answered. Miller obviously hoped that aid to European scientists would continue unabated, and he was eager to present what he perceived as an exciting prospect.

The formal proposal, consisting of three parts written by both Florey and Chain, was mailed on November 20 to both Paris and New York. Florey recounted the ingenuity and achievements of his staff since the last Rockefeller grant in 1936, three years before. Chain crafted a section entitled "A Chemical Study of the Phenomenon of Bacterial Antagonism." He added that antibacterial properties of such substances as lysozyme and "the mould penicillium notatum" suggested that "they seem therefore to possess great potentialities for therapeutic application."

The program of research was not limited to bacterial antagonism; in keeping with his long-standing research into mucus, Florey added a section on it. Then Florey did the numbers: £5,000 spread over three years (or about $20,000). This allowed for £1,670 in wages for two technical assistants, a mechanic, and a "fully qualified biochemist"; another £500 a year was for laboratory supplies. Florey included an additional request not to exceed £1,000 to buy "non-recurring" equipment that ranged from a £150 "Step photometer" to a £10 "Ice-crushing machine" and a £5 "Volt-amp meter," explaining, "It has often taken months to get special pieces of apparatus owing to the necessity of approaching outside bodies, the trustees of which meet at long intervals, for relatively small sums of money."

The foundation approved the request for a year but with the expectation that it would be renewed twice. Because of internal restrictions on grants of this nature, the most that could be awarded per year was $5,000, or £1,250. This was more than compensated for by the grant actually being approved for up to five years (although Florey was not immediately told this), barring severe interruption of the work by the war. On February 19, 1940, Miller informed Florey that the first year's money "for the important research . . . under your direction" would be available on March 1.

Florey, Chain, and the others at the Dunn School reacted as if they had won the lottery, which, insofar as scientific funding went, they had. Florey thanked Miller for his "magnificent assistance." This was support on a grand scale and it meant that for the first time his team would not have to chase after many small grants to cobble together a research program. The news made the usually reserved Florey ebullient. He and Chain had a celebration in Chain's flat, along with Anna Sacharina and a visiting friend of Chain's.

This grant did not mean the end of other work by the Dunn School staff. In October 1939, the MRC asked Florey to direct a research program on shock, an often-fatal complication from serious injury. Little was understood about it, including so simple a point as whether its onset is accompanied by high blood pressure. (It is not.) With the prospect of massive battlefield and air-raid casualties, more information was desperately needed. In a piece of great good fortune for the work on penicillin, Dr. Edward Abraham, a chemist on a Rockefeller fellowship in Stockholm, cut short his stay and returned to England in November. He had been on Robert Robinson's staff at the Dyson Perrins Lab, doing work on lysozyme and then on a protein project, and he hoped he could resume that research. The project had been abandoned, however, and Robinson suggested that Abraham join Florey and Chain on the wound shock project. Abraham had first met Chain, briefly, in 1938 for a discussion on lysozyme. His "sole abiding memory of that occasion" was that Chain "was very different from anyone I had met before." Florey was able to get Abraham an MRC grant. Soon he was enmeshed in the chemical work on penicillin and would be instrumental in deciphering its makeup.

There were other consequences of war, among them the evacuation of people, children especially, from areas thought to be in greatest danger of air raids. Charles and Paquita Florey were sent to Cornwall for safety, then, in an instance of curious bureaucratic logic, six children and two teachers from London took their rooms in Oxford. Gordon Sanders dropped by the house one day to find Ethel dividing a large mattress in two with a saw.

The work on penicillin went into high gear when Heatley joined in the work and took over the growing of the mold in its shallow liquid medium.

At first, the experiments used between fifty and a hundred liters a week of medium. Experiments showed that the ideal depth for the best yield was no more than 1.5 cm. The fronds, or mycelium, of greenish-blue mold fluffed above the surface and dropped spores that planted the seeds for more mold. In time, yellowish gold droplets rich in penicillin formed on the dry mycelium and were drawn off by a pipette to be tested. The medium also turned yellow as penicillin settled into it. Within a few months, Heatley would discover that if the penicillin-rich fluid in the medium under the mold were drawn off when it reached its highest concentration, and then fresh medium put in its place, penicillin could be grown not only faster but with less effort, and that this could be repeated up to fourteen times before starting again by incubating a fresh layer of mold. Eventually, however, a troublesome spore-bearing organism that insinuated itself in the mold caused so much contamination that the procedure was abandoned, and each dish of medium and mold used only once.

There were, Florey reasoned, four interlocking puzzles to solve: How to grow the most and the most potent mold; which bacteria were affected by penicillin and to what degree; what, if any, were the effects on human cells and tissues; and what were penicillin's chemical structure and the means of its action?

At this stage of the investigation, when the difficulties in producing penicillin precluded solving the biological and bacteriological problems, no one at the Dunn School was more needed or more useful than Heatley. "He was a most versatile, ingenious, and skilled laboratory engineer on any scale, large or minute," Gwyn Macfarlane wrote of his friend. "To his training in biology and biochemistry he could add the technical skills of optics, glass- and metal-working, plumbing, carpentry, and as much electrical work as was needed in those pre-electronic days. Above all, he could improvise—making use of the most unlikely bits of laboratory or household equipment to do a job with the least possible waste of time."

One of Heatley's first tasks was to find a more productive means of growing the mold, which, to him, meant starting at the beginning. "The only practical information Chain passed on to the person who was taking over from him (i.e. me)," he wrote thirty-five years later, "was a very quaint method of sowing the broth in a pie dish. Only two pie dishes were handed over, again suggesting very little was done" prior to September 1939. Heatley immediately set his mind to the problem, as well as to that of devising a better method for testing the potency of each batch of penicillin.

Finding a quick way to assay the activity of a substance is one of the first hurdles to cross in the investigation of any biological material whose nature is yet unknown, because it is through the biological effects alone that its potency or concentration can be measured. The way to make that measurement is to test the strength of the substance at various times in its production against a single organism. It is rather like a cook preparing a new dish several ways, trying to find the best combination of ingredients and cooking time. Assay tests determine the ideal recipe and cooking time, and they can be done by either dilution or diffusion.

In dilution, a specific amount is mixed with sterile water in a measured way, testing it first at full strength and then, say, at one part in ten, one part in one thousand, and so on, until there is no discernible effect. The stronger the original solution, the more it can be diluted and still be effective. This method leads to an answer, but it is also time-consuming and requires complete sterilization at every stage to prevent contamination from skewing the results.

Diffusion is simpler. A petri dish is seeded with bacteria, a drop of the antibacterial substance being assayed is put on it, and the dish is incubated overnight. By the next morning, bacterial growth will cover the plate, except—as Fleming's contaminated dish showed—for the clear circles where the antibiotic reaction has occurred; the bigger the circle, the stronger the solution.

The method Heatley used for penicillin was based on a technique of Florey's, in which holes were drilled in the bottom of a petri dish and then closed with rubber stoppers. A waxy agar medium was poured into the dishes, and, when it had set, the plate was turned over and the stoppers removed, leaving small cuplike indentations. Whatever fluid was to be tested was poured into the little cups of agar and then incubated so the bacteria could grow, like a hen warming her eggs. The active material divided and diffused through the agar; the further it diffused, the stronger it was.

Heatley reasoned that penicillin should do the same thing, and it did, but the large size of the holes combined with what Heatley described as not "the best sort of glass and equipment" made precise measurement difficult. After just three days on the job, Heatley realized that by using small Pyrex glass tubes as cylinders planted in the agar, diffusion could be measured more quickly and with greater accuracy. A short while later he replaced the Pyrex cylinders with others made of porcelain.

Heatley's new idea vastly improved the way penicillin was assayed. Current practice was to use a dilution test, which Heatley found to be "an awful bother. If your sample is not sterile, you can't do a dilution test because anything will grow and you'll get quite erratic results." Even sterilizing a sample and then doing a dilution test is not a very precise measure. All one can learn is that this solution inhibited a certain species of staphylococcus at a dilution of one in one hundred but it didn't at one in two hundred. That is a cumbersome way of measuring the strength of one batch against another, and so, after Heatley solved the problem of preserving the activity of penicillin once it was extracted, in March 1940, Heatley and Florey agreed to establish an arbitrary standard solution.

Heatley's diary for October 1939 details his many ideas for and success in assaying penicillin, which was not yet a catchword and whose spelling varied. "Quite encouraging results from the penecillin [sic] testing technique," he noted with pleasure at the end of his first week on the job. His plate and cylinder assay allowed for quick and simple identification of results. Half a dozen or so cylinders were inserted into each plate of agar sowed with Staphylococcus aureus. In usual practice, petri dishes are covered with a glass top and turned upside down so that moisture will not condense on the top during incubation, then drip into the culture and contaminate it. Turning over the cylinders, however, would have spilled the penicillin. Heatley realized that if he rested the bottoms of the dishes on wood strips rather than directly on the shelves, air would circulate and prevent condensation. After incubation for twelve to sixteen hours, the plate was set over a glass ruler lit from beneath and the size of the growth-free circle around the cylinder was recorded.

(Florey would improve this method in 1942 when he discovered that the cylinders would more firmly fuse and be less prone to leaking if they were first heated—but not too much—in a flame and then plunged into the agar. "The noise accompanying the operation should be a short 'psst!' rather than a prolonged sizzle," he cautioned. As the pace of the development of antibiotics quickened over the next decade, Heatley's plate and cylinder process would be used hundreds of millions of times by scientists around the world.)

While Heatley worked at getting the mold to grow more quickly and produce more penicillin, Chain concentrated on the biochemical problems of purifying and isolating its antibacterial element. One of his first discoveries was that whatever this element was, it passed easily through the tiny pores of a cellophane filter. Even though cellophane seems nonporous, on a chemical level it is a sieve; chemistry works on a *very* small scale, and physics on an even smaller one.

So despite every assumption, penicillin was far too small and simple a molecule to be an enzyme. This only further complicated the puzzle because penicillin's instability—its antibacterial effect vanished during extraction—meant that neither could it be a protein.

Chain, initially sure that penicillin was an enzyme, naturally was at first disappointed as "my beautiful working hypothesis dissolved into thin air." At the same time, "it became very interesting to find out which structural features were responsible for the instability. It was clear that we were dealing with a chemically very unusual substance." This, however, changed the basic nature of the problem he was trying to solve. "Instead of studying the isolation and mode of action of an enzyme with strong antibacterial properties, our task was now the elucidation of the structure of a low molecular substance which combined high antibacterial power with great chemical instability." Which meant their task was on the order of finding an Abominable Snowman who also tap-danced.

Unlike Raistrick, who when confronted by penicillin's instability simply gave up on it, Chain was now more fascinated than ever. Like Raistrick, Chain at least partially purified penicillin by mixing it with water to dissolve it and then mixing it with ether. The ether captured the soluble penicillin but left the generally insoluble impurities intact and thus easy to discard. But then the penicillin vanished as it was removed from the ether.

Captivated by penicillin's inherent instability, Chain tested its stability at varying pH levels and found that it was stable only at the edges of acid and basic, from pH5 to pH8; pure water—pH7—is neutral. He also learned that extraction at the freezing point maintained more of penicillin's activity, and that by frequently adding alkali to nudge the acidic mixture back to neutral, he could get most of this active penicillin back into water. It was like herding butterflies. That still left him with the problem of how to dry or crystallize penicillin without destroying it.

Meanwhile, in his search for the medium that would grow the most potent penicillin in the shortest time, Heatley tinkered with the broth in which the mold grew as if making soup for a finicky child, recording in black ink in his lab book the precise details of every ingredient and jotting pertinent notes beside them in red. He added nitrate, sodium, and aluminum salts; he put in glucose (a sugar); he mixed sucrose (another sugar) and lactate (an acid) with a reduction of cow and horse muscle; he tried extracts of malt and of various meats; he variously stirred in greater and lesser amounts of phosphate (a salt of phosphoric acid), glycerol (a soluble alcohol), peptone (a protein), oxygen, and carbon dioxide; he even slipped in some Marmite, the sticky, salty, brown yeast-based spread that is to some English and Australians ambrosia and to most of the world anathema. He noted the effect of each on how the mold grew and behaved, and all he learned was that none of the recipes he concocted were helpful.

Sometimes, even though to all appearances the mold grew normally and the broth turned yellow, no penicillin at all was produced. The obvious conclusion was that contamination had crept in, but that proved not to be the case. Instead, Heatley found that some of the mold simply did not produce penicillin, and, if inactive spores were seeded, there would be no yield. Eventually Heatley kept what amounted to a starter colony by selecting spores from batches that produced the greatest amount of penicillin and used it to grow his cultures. Because of this and the search for the right recipe, in the early going, Chain was fortunate when he had a milligram—one twenty-eight-thousandth of an ounce—to work with at any one time. By the middle of March 1940, however, Heatley was able to provide Chain with close to 100 mg for his experiments.

Just before Christmas 1939, Florey had a visit from an old friend and colleague who in conversation with Heatley suggested that perhaps yeast would help speed the fermenting of the mold juice. Heatley went to Morrell's, a local brewery, and got some. Yeast extract cut the fermentation time in half, to ten days. However, it did not improve the yield.

Neither was Heatley and Chain's relationship much improved. Although Heatley was happier now that he reported directly to Florey, his difficulties in working with Chain continued. He later wrote:

> [Our] increasing friction was, of course, a reflection of my own character, and was built on hundreds of trivial incidents. . . . [Chain] often expected unquestioning agreement with his views . . . and this was sometimes carried to absurd lengths. Example: Till 1942 or later all samples of penicillin were yellow. A yellow pigment could easily be separated from it. In 1940 or '41 EC said that penicillin itself was yellow. I replied that it might be, but that there was no evidence that it was. EC replied 'Heatley, I am *telling* you that it is yellow. Yellow! Yellow!!' Penicillin was later found to be colourless. Why did arguments of this sort go on for half an hour, sometimes? EC was no doubt trying to insist on the Teutonic convention that the Geheimrat's authority was absolute; on my side, I refused—perhaps too obstinately—to agree to a postulate I knew was untrue. There were also many arguments where we held different, but at the time valid, views . . . but they dragged on and wasted a lot of nervous energy. I was irritated, too, that these discussions started just as I was beginning or about to begin my picnic lunch in my room.

The lab day followed a routine that began with everyone's arrival around nine A.M. Lunch, almost always at one's workbench, was at about one. There was a break for tea in the main lab in the afternoon, with talk often entirely about trivial things. Around six P.M. everyone went home, although sometimes an experiment required monitoring after dinner. Florey usually joined the other professors of Lincoln College for dinner at the high table in the college dining hall while Ethel and the children ate at home.

In early February, Chain asked Heatley if he would like to work with him and another scientist on a new freezing-drying apparatus they were going to build. "I had leaped at the idea," he wrote in his diary, "but last night after turning it over for a long time I thought there would only be trouble if Chain and I collaborated, so this morning I told Chain I was not so keen. This did not seem to worry him much."

A couple of weeks later came evidence of why he was right not to join the collaboration. "On arrival at the lab found that the penicillin which had been distilling yesterday had evaporated to dryness and distilled all night. Stormy scene with Chain in which he tended to blame *me* for it." Their mutual grating continued. "P is slightly absorbed by charcoal at acid PH, or it may be destroyed," he noted in mid-March after carrying out an experiment that paralleled work Chain was doing. "Had a row with Chain because he objects to me doing his work, or rather not telling him about it. He was quite right in a way."

All of which may help explain why Chain dismissed an idea Heatley had on March 18, 1940, that would turn out to greatly advance their work. "Had a discussion with the Professor and Chain about the future of the penicillin work," is all Heatley recorded in his diary. Conferences like this with Florey were a rarity. Florey's style was to let scientists do their work without interference or mass meetings. This did not mean he was unaware of what was going on in the various lab rooms; in fact, most days he would stop by each person's workbench and chat about experiments in progress. Suggestions made in passing as he left often led to useful progress.

Practicality was Florey's hallmark; "Do the experiment" his motto. According to Henry Harris, he

genuinely disliked theory. The scientists whom he admired were those who had done practical things, who had made discoveries that produce visible effects on people's lives. If, in discussing your work with him . . . you began to speculate, his eyes would glaze over and it was clear that he had stopped listening. . . . The other side of the coin was that Florey's no-nonsense approach to science rubbed off on us all. No one who ever worked with him or under his direction remained unmarked by the experience. We all adopted his astringent criteria of what was a good experiment and what wasn't; we all tried to devise simple direct approaches to our problems; we didn't seek to inflate the importance of our work by showmanship or self-advertisement; and when we talked about experiments we told the truth.

The discussion with Chain and Heatley centered on why so far it was impossible to extract penicillin from the ether solution without its vanishing in the process. There had to be a way to get it out and keep it effective, Florey said again and again as he and Chain did most of the talking and Heatley mainly listened. When Heatley finally did speak, he seemed half apologetic for putting forward what he later called a "laughably simple" idea that had heretofore crossed no one's mind.

His idea was to use a chemical yo-yo, a notion along the lines of Isaac Newton's principle that for every action there is an equal and opposite reaction. If penicillin could be extracted from a neutral buffer of water into ether, why shouldn't it be possible to transfer it out of the ether into water made alkaline?

Florey was intrigued by the idea, but, according to Heatley, Chain characterized the deduction as "unsound." After some additional wrangling with Florey, whose enthusiasm was unshaken, Heatley recorded that Chain realized the argument was lost, and with a shrug told him, "Then if you think it will work, why don't you do it yourself? That will surely be the best and quickest way to show that you are wrong."

Chain later wrote that what Florey and Heatley interpreted as Chain's dismissal of Heatley's idea was merely a gesture of irritation that they were usurping his work. "I must state categorically that I never said . . . that Heatley's experiments would [not] work, and have never been able to understand on what basis and at what time this story was invented." On several occasions in the years to come, Florey, whose recollection matched Heatley's, told Heatley that he wished the conversation had been tape-recorded so that Chain's claim might be deflated.

Chain's version of the meeting was that reverse extraction "may be a good idea but it was chemical work in which I was fully involved, and [I] reminded Florey and Heatley that we had agreed that the chemical work would be done by myself. Therefore, I asked, why not let me continue what I was already doing? Florey . . . [said] that in any case it did not matter who did what at this stage as everything would be published jointly."

The underlying issue for Chain was that he viewed Florey's turning extraction over to Heatley as a betrayal. Heatley's clear brief was production while Chain's was to deal with the chemical problems. Extraction could have fallen into either category. The nub of Chain's unhappiness was quite likely in the difference between his view and Florey's of how a laboratory should be run. Florey's encouragement of a workplace with a free-flowing intellectual intercourse did not imply that everyone was equal, but it did mean that everyone should be heard and that work could be shared. He felt good work would always be acknowledged (he would be disappointed on this score in later years). To Chain, once the tasks were confused, it was difficult to tell who was in charge and to whom credit should go, and it was important that proper credit be given him. Perhaps his immigrant status fostered that.

Thus, even though Heatley is the one who solved the riddle of penicillin's instability, Chain felt cheated.

> This was once again a clear breach of an agreement between Florey and myself and I expressed with a gesture my disappointment and annoyance that one could not trust any undertaking given by Florey. I gave in in the end, because I could not afford a serious row at that stage because of my special position in the country which was very weak. I had become a naturalized British citizen just a few months before this conversation took place and had to avoid any action which could provoke latent anti-Semitism which was very widespread. I had to bear in mind the fact that the Jewish community would not be very pleased if controversies of any kind with anti-Semitic undertones came into the open. Florey knew of my weak position and exploited it repeatedly; he also knew that he would find support in any action he took by the then secretary of the MRC, Mellanby.

While in retrospect this incident may seem blown out of proportion, it is the accumulation of slights, real or perceived, that can poison any relationship. It also demonstrates the creeping dissonance in a trio whose attention was concentrated on a single goal that required all their talents. There is no doubt that Chain's fears were deeply felt, but it is difficult to see anti-Semitism on Florey's part. He enthusiastically hired Chain; he applauded the work he did on lysozyme; in their walks to and from work, he displayed more openness and friendship than he showed to anyone else in the lab; and he entrusted Chain to write a critical part of the proposal to the Rockefeller Foundation, on which their joint futures hung. Yet even after his permanent scientific honor was secured, Chain's sense of injustice not only remained, it was amplified; he carried it until his death in 1979. (Henry Harris feels that anti-Semitism played no part in "anything that happened—or not—to Chain. . . . I just think that his demeanor got on everyone's nerves because he was so immensely conceited.")

Heatley immediately set to work to test what he proposed. He knew that to achieve separation he needed to use two solutions that would not mix, so that each could do its particular chemical job. The transfer depended on penicillin turning out to be an acid, which is more soluble in organic solutions such as ether or amyl acetate than it is in water.

On March 19, he filtered acidified mold juice through some surplus parachute silk to weed out bits of mold and other trash, mixed the filtrate with ether, and shook it; then he let the liquid sit to allow the lighter ether (now containing the penicillin) to rise and form the top layer. The heavier water beneath it was drained off through a separating funnel. He put the remaining ether/penicillin in a jar with some alkaline water and shook this mixture. Just as he suspected, the penicillin, now extracted from both the mold juice and the ether, passed back into water—without disappearing. Another experiment done on March 20 showed an even clearer result. The back-extracted neutral watery solution showed no loss of activity after eleven days at room temperature. This stability meant it was likely that a drug from penicillin could be easily transported and stored, essential for potential medical applications.

Twelve years after Fleming first saw penicillin's disappearing act, there was now a way to keep it in view. Ironically, by this time, Fleming was involved in studying the sulfonamides; four of his five papers published in 1940 were on them or on antiseptics.

Extraction had to be carried out at low temperatures to help stabilize the penicillin in its acidified stage. The Oxford group knew from Fleming's work that heat destroyed it, and from Raistrick's experiments that it could be kept stable in an ice box for three months.

Work by Chain in early 1940 confirmed earlier observations that if penicillin were kept cool, it would not immediately disappear.

The extraction had to be done in the lab's six-foot-square cold room, which, since it was just above freezing, was an obviously uncomfortable environment for a technician. Heatley spent considerable time in refrigerated surroundings doing the early extraction work, and, on at least one winter's day when doing an experiment to find the optimum temperature for extraction, he put on gloves, an overcoat, and scarf, and took the large bottles of extract and ether onto the snow-covered roof of the Dunn School, where he rocked the bottles back and forth to coax out the penicillin.

From the spring of 1940 into early 1941, Heatley devised and refined an automated extraction apparatus, called a countercurrent machine. Rube Goldberg and his British counterpart W. Heath Robinson would have envied the device, which required several modifications and revampings before it worked properly. His first design included a fifteen-foot-long piece of spiraled glass he had flattened. The final model, whose frame he made after demolishing a discarded oak bookcase from the Bodleian Library, was about six feet high and three feet wide. It consisted of glass tubing mostly made by Heatley, assorted pumps, laboratory bottles, an old doorbell to signal when a bottle was about to become empty or full, colored warning lights, nozzles, copper cooling coils that he fashioned, and more junctions between the various bottles and tubes than on the track of a complex electric train set. Altogether it might have cost £5. The machine was used until November 1941, but unfortunately none of it has survived. One historian has likened it to "Röntgen's original X-ray tube or Lister's first air-sterilization plant designed to effect asepsis in the operating theatre." In the 1980s, the Science Museum asked Heatley to build a replica, which he found more expensive to assemble. "The rubbish dumps aren't what they were in the 1940s," he said.

Heatley's ability to construct from virtually nothing all that his mind envisioned is a trait common to some of the most innovative scientists. Certainly Fleming would have admired such industry. As the scientist and historian Robert Scott Root-Bernstein points out, Pasteur made his own apparatus. Frederick Banting and Charles H. Best, the Canadians who isolated insulin in 1921, had no academic position and no salary when they made their breakthrough. The research performed in Cambridge University's Cavendish Laboratory when it was led between 1919 and 1937 by Ernest Rutherford (the father of nuclear physics) was usually done on a mélange of thickly cut pine or fir tables pushed together to create a work space littered with equipment cobbled together from odd bits and imagination. Charles T. R. Wilson, one of the most creative members of the Cavendish, supposedly never spent more than £5 on an instrument. (The Wilson diffusion cloud chamber allowed for the first photographs of the movement of electrons, in 1896.) J. F. Adolf von Baeyer (pioneering work on dyestuffs and carbon rings), John William Strutt, Lord Rayleigh (who discovered the inert gas argon in 1895 and whose 1871 theory of scattering explained why the sky is blue), and Wilhelm Röntgen (X-rays, 1895) all produced their spectacular results on inexpensive and self-assembled equipment. Ernest O. Lawrence built the first subatomic particle accelerator, or cyclotron, in 1929, in Berkeley, California, for a few dollars, and his second version for under a hundred. The German Otto Hahn split the atom in 1938 with a machine he made from easily available parts and that fit on a desktop. Each of these scientists won a Nobel Prize.

The countercurrent machine duplicated Heatley's original extraction process, but it did so continuously and on a greater scale. The more the details of its construction, the less understandable it becomes, even though his underlying theory was simple: Two liquids of different molecular weights will settle into two distinct layers after being mixed, like oil and water.

Three one-gallon bottles each of cooled filtrate, ether, and acid were turned upside down into a frame built atop the bookshelf; a bung designed by Heatley kept the contents in until, once in place, a slight downward push moved aside a glass ball stopper.

The bottles emptied into a cooling coil surrounded by ice. Glass tubes were connected through stoppers in the necks that allowed the brew to be acidified with phosphoric acid just before it was jet-sprayed into a tube.

The drops had to be a certain size: too big and they ran together;

too small and they sank slowly and flooded the apparatus. Getting the right-sized jets proved difficult; a variety of handmade glass and metal ones failed. Finally, in a perfect example of his skill at microscales, Heatley embedded the point of a needle in a piece of hot glass to make a punch of the exact width he wanted. After it cooled, he used it to puncture uniform holes in a platinum disk at specific points.

Now the hard part. Once collected, the acidified filtrate flowed down one of six parallel separation tubes; ether was released from the bottom and flowed past it in the four-foot-long tubes that separated the bottles. The filtrate was then sprayed into a tube of rising ether continually fed in from the bottom. Because penicillin has a greater affinity for ether than it does for the broth in which it grows, it transferred when the two were mixed. The heavy impurities from the filtrate sank and were drained out at the bottom while the penicillin/acetate compound rose and was collected in a bottle that was removed by hand when it was full.

The same counterflow method was used to retrieve the penicillin from the acidified acetate or ether. The rising penicillin was captured from the ether by descending water made slightly alkaline. The mixture of penicillin and water (now about one-fifth of what it was at the start) was drawn off at the bottom and then purified. The solvent was returned to the first stage. After distillation in a steam-heated zinc trash can devised by Heatley to remove any bits of water, the ether was used again and again. (Ether is highly inflammable, but as it was the only solvent known to extract penicillin, the risk was necessary. Then one day Chain suggested trying amyl acetate, which worked equally well and was less flammable; even though it had its own side effects, such as causing anemia, it was used from then on, leaving a telltale scent of pears.)

Heatley's countercurrent machine could process twelve liters of crude broth per hour, though not without difficulty. "In the opinion of some at least of those who used it," Florey wrote, "it was almost as temperamental as a prima donna. Nevertheless . . . it gave valuable service."

Next came the need to purify the penicillin and store it while preserving its activity. Freeze-drying was devised by Swedish chemists in 1935 but did not come into great use until after the start of the war, when it made necessities such as blood plasma and milk easy to store and transport. Because freeze-drying can produce enzymes without affecting their potency, Chain was correct in postulating that this method would maintain the activity of penicillin. The end result, he later wrote, was "a very nice brown powder which kept the activity of the medium undiminished, without any loss whatsoever." The powder was so strong—it prevented bacterial growth when diluted to one part in a million and was twenty times greater than any sulphonamide—that at first everyone in the lab presumed it must have been quite pure. In fact, it contained about thirty different substances.

Heatley, meanwhile, continued his experiments with extraction and what effect various compounds had on penicillin and recorded the results in his diary. "Tried incubating P with rat blood and rat liver," he wrote on March 28; the penicillin was not destroyed. (Heatley once greeted some lab workers he encountered in the hall with lines from the witches' feast in *Macbeth*: "Fillet of a fenny snake, / In the cauldron boil and bake. / Eye of newt and toe of frog, / Wool of bat and tongue of dog. . . .")

In counterpoint to this fine scientific progress, Chain and Florey's personal relations continued to fray. According to a 1979 letter from Chain to Gwyn Macfarlane, during February and March 1940, he went to Florey at least four times to ask him to perform a toxicity test of penicillin on a lab animal.

> The last time I appeared in his laboratory with this request, Florey turned to Mrs. M. Jennings (who was standing next to Sanders engaged with Florey in attempts to extirpate lymph nodes from rats in order to understand the function of lymphocytes) saying, pointing to me, "In one of my weak moments I promised this man to test his fractions and here he comes pestering me again." After these humiliating remarks in front of others not involved in the project it became clear to me that Florey was not really interested in penicillin and I decided to ask my friend Barnes to do the first preliminary experiments.

The incident highlights the personality of each man, one working enthusiastically on a specific project, the other running a whole department and conducting other experiments as well. As Chain's biographer Ronald Clark put it, "Florey sometimes threw off casual remarks without appreciating the seriousness with which others take them [and] Chain . . . was at times unable to consider such a remark as anything less than a seriously planned attempt to score off him."

Chain was hardly being singled out; Florey's remark was wholly in character, and its style completely predictable. Since his school days in Australia, he had been unable to praise himself or anyone else, at least to their face. "We seem to be shuffling our feet," was a common piece of Floriana, and often the most enthusiasm he could show for a proposed piece of work was, "Well it seems we won't be doing any harm." Henry Harris suffered the fate of everyone who worked with Florey:

Although he was obviously interested in what I was doing, his overt reaction was always disparagement. If he came back to Oxford after an absence abroad and I chanced to cross him in the corridor, his greeting would always be a disparaging remark. "Ah there, Harris, still going backwards?" or perhaps, "Ah there, Harris, made any discoveries lately?" I naturally found all this cold water rather depressing until I learned by chance that while he was disparaging me to my face he was singing my praises elsewhere. . . . After that I was perfectly happy to take as much disparagement as Florey was prepared to dish out, but some of the young men working in the department reacted very differently. Florey's cold style drove them to despair.

After one young scientist won a prestigious award, Florey congratulated him and then quickly added, "Of course, there happened to be a poor field this year."

In regard to the more critical detail of Florey's supposed lack of interest, Heatley's diary for this period is filled with references to Florey's almost daily involvement in the penicillin work. Still, Chain's feeling was as sincere as his enthusiasm was unbridled, and undoubtedly he felt that his work was not receiving the attention that to him it deserved.

———

In order to perform animal tests, a scientist needed a special license from the Home Office, which Chain did not have. Dr. John M. Barnes did. A member of the Dunn School staff but not one of those working on penicillin, he already was doing injections for Chain on another project. Reports differ as to exactly how much penicillin was tested, but Chain dissolved in 2 ml (.06 ounces) of water between 40 and 80 ml (.001 to .002 ounces) of penicillin—roughly between 40 and 80 percent of all the penicillin on hand—and on March 19, Barnes injected the abdominal lining of each of two mice with 1 ml of the mixture.

Nothing happened. There was no reaction at all, at least in the mice. Chain, however, was elated. To him, "this was the crucial day in the whole development . . . of penicillin. . . . Why this simple extraction and toxicity had not been done before is difficult to say."

Just why he felt that way is unclear, since Fleming achieved the same result (but with a smaller dose) on a mouse and a rabbit in 1929, and Florey had stated quite plainly in his application to Rockefeller that penicillin was "non-toxic to animals, even in large doses." All Chain's test really showed was that penicillin of uncertain purity—the powder he used had not been assayed—in this specific preparation was not toxic.

But these tests did grab Florey's attention, if only because it was he and not Chain who was in charge of the biological testing. When Florey reminded Chain of this, Chain pointed out that "you were too busy with other work."

"This will be different in the future," Chain says Florey vowed.

However great the misunderstandings, what really matters is that these tests led to a crucial discovery.

Florey, his attention focused and perhaps his pride wounded, was determined to do a toxicity test on a mouse himself with the remaining penicillin. There was just one problem: for all his vast experience with conducting tests on animals, Florey had never needed to know how to inject into the vein of a mouse. His counterpart in pharmacology, Professor J. H. Burn, gave him a quick lesson. Once tutored, Florey injected approximately 20 ml of penicillin into the tail vein and saw for himself that there was no toxicity. According to the still-aggrieved Chain, "He was so skeptical about this that he thought he had missed the vein," and wanted to repeat the experiment. Soon some additional penicillin was produced that, when injected, caused no damage in the mouse.

However, there was an unmistakable sign that Florey had indeed hit the vein and that the brown pigment of the injected penicillin had passed through the kidneys of the mouse: when Florey turned the animal over, there was a pool of deep brown urine. This was not a complete surprise as the pigment had also passed through the extraction process. But what had become of the active ingredient in the penicillin? Chain and Florey placed a drop of the urine on an agar plate and found that it had an enormous antibacterial power.

Chain immediately grasped the implication: "We knew then that here we had a substance that was non-toxic, and not destroyed in the body and therefore was certain to act against bacteria *in vivo*."

Penicillin suddenly looked not only like an interesting chemical, it looked like a drug.

7

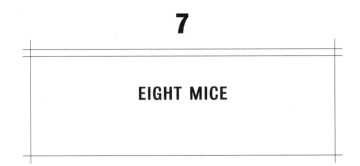

EIGHT MICE

The race was on. Penicillin was no longer a chemical and biological abstraction. Now it had the potential to save many of the hundreds of British lives that were being lost every day.

During April and May 1940, Florey, Margaret Jennings, and James Kent carried out precise experiments on cats, rats, rabbits, and mice to quantify exactly how penicillin was absorbed and excreted and what, if any, toxicity it possessed. Fortunately, they did not try it on guinea pigs, the one rodent that reacts badly to penicillin: the drug kills penicillin-sensitive bacteria in the intestine, which are quickly replaced by other bacteria that help absorb toxins and lead to blood poisoning. If they had, the work would have been set back considerably.

One major question was how best to administer penicillin so that the maximum amount of the antibiotic was absorbed by the body. They gave penicillin orally, and via a tube into the stomach; in each case stomach acid destroyed it. However, it was absorbed unharmed when administered by a tube into the duodenum, just below the stomach and the shortest, widest, and most fixed part of the small intestine. Penicillin was injected intravenously, directly into the bloodstream. It was injected into the peritoneum, the meshlike membrane that lines the abdominal wall, in order to diffuse the dose. And it was injected subcutaneously, just beneath the skin. All methods of injection allowed the drug to do its work. But within an hour or two, the penicillin was virtually gone from the blood, a sign that it had lost its effectiveness or had been excreted. This meant that it had to be readministered frequently, thus requiring more precious penicillin. Because the urine of injected mice turned brown, it was evident that the bulk of the penicillin was being passed unchanged through the kidneys. The unused penicillin was extracted from the urine and reused.

Toxicity was an obvious concern. For all the promise the sulfonamides initially offered, they were often effective against disease only at the point that the dose became poisonous to the patient, hardly ideal for a medicine. If penicillin would prove equally compromised, a good way to check was to determine how white blood cells were affected by it. White blood cells, or leucocytes, which help fight infection, are excellent indicators of toxicity: if they've been killed, they can't fight. They have the added value of being easily studied in a test tube. Florey's former colleague at Sheffield Cecil G. Paine had already done work on the effect of sulfonamides on leucocytes, and so Florey asked him for the details of his procedures and adjusted them for working with penicillin.

The results were stunning. Even when penicillin was diluted to one part per million it killed bacteria, yet in a solution of one in five hundred (two thousand times stronger), it had no effect on white cells. Peter Medawar, the future Nobel Prize winner for his part in the discovery of acquired immunological intolerance, carried the tests further by looking for ill effect on tissue cells that were growing; these, too, proved unharmed. Margaret Jennings then took over his work.

While these tests were conducted, Florey's colleagues Duncan Gardner and Jean Orr-Ewing tested penicillin against the microbes most troublesome to humans. In carefully observing these microbes as they grew—or failed to grow—in petri dishes where penicillin was present, Gardner confirmed that penicillin was neither an enzyme that dissolved cells nor an antiseptic that killed them. Rather, the microbes swelled and elongated, but, instead of dividing, as they must do to reproduce, they exploded or simply died. Gardner reported in *Nature* that sublethal doses of penicillin caused stunning changes in the cells that survived: they became grossly swollen and their rods grew eight or ten times, and sometimes even thirty times, their normal length.

In the same issue of *Nature,* Chain and Abraham reported that certain contaminants in the mold broth spurred production of penicillinaise, an enzyme that destroys penicillin. In years to come, this finding would have great significance.

When penicillin worked, however, something in it prevented cell division. Whatever caused that debilitating effect on basic bacterial function allowed penicillin to act against a wide range of bacteria that cause disease.

Unfortunately, one of those diseases was not tuberculosis. This was a major disappointment to Gardner and the others because, at the time, tuberculosis killed thirty thousand Britons each year and destroyed the health of hundreds of thousands more; in the years following World War II, TB was probably the most widespread disease in the world, responsible for around 3.5 million deaths a year. (It is still a deadly menace, killing about 2 million people per year—more than two hundred every hour.)

However, this failure was more than compensated for by penicillin's effectiveness against (in descending order of strength) the bacteria that cause gonorrhea and meningitis; infections caused by staphylococcus, then streptococcus; followed by those that cause anthrax, lumpy abscesses, tetanus, gas gangrene, lobar pneumonia, and diphtheria. Moreover, unlike the sulfonamides, penicillin worked in wounds where there was pus and other fluids and in tissue that was breaking down from infection.

These were tremendously exciting findings, but the biggest question was still to be answered.

Penicillin clearly worked in the test tube. But it remained to be seen if it worked in a living animal, a much more complex proving ground where unknown factors could render penicillin worthless, or provide immunity to it. If the tests showed an equal effectiveness in the body, human life would be fundamentally changed; diseases and infections that had forever been a scourge to humans would suddenly be conquerable. Put simply, a scratch from a rose thorn need no longer lead to death.

All this took place as it became ever more evident that the war could come to British soil. On May 13, 1940, "a gloriously fine sunny day," Heatley noted that he "spent all morning, with most of the other people at the lab, filling sandbags from a pile of earth close to the observatory," then bringing them to the Dunn School and stacking them into air-raid shelters. Beginning on May 20, four people spent the night at the lab to keep guard over it in case of fire from bombing. Heatley devoted much of whatever free time he had to work with scientists at a defense firm on an engineering problem with a bubble sextant used for aerial navigation, and from May 1940 until the next spring, he spent most Saturday afternoons taking blood from donors at a nearby hospital.

Between his own defense chores, Duncan Gardner was asked to prepare a test batch of streptococcus that would be injected into mice, which would then receive penicillin. It was not that easy a task.

"I had to do many carefully quantitative tests," he later wrote, "to determine the exact dose which would just, and only just, kill a mouse of normal weight in 24 to 36 hours (too big a dose would not give the penicillin a proper chance)." And not just one mouse, but also whatever number of mice of normal weight that were to be used in any experiment; no mouse should be left alive because it overcame the infection on its own. Calibrating the right dose posed additional obstacles for Gardner. "The whole affair was rather tricky, as cultures of microbes have to be re-cultured daily, and are capable of varying a lot from day to day in virulence and other properties. So my final tests had to be done or repeated just before the culture was to be used in the chemotherapeutic experiment, and quite a lot of mice had to be used. The whole experiment depended on getting the dose right."

Gardner chose for the tests a strain called *Streptococcus haemolyticus*, a microbe "I used to call public enemy number one, as it was the cause of more severe and fatal infections than any other single species: puerperal fever, septicemia, meningitis, erysipelas [a painful and infectious skin disease] and scarlet fever."

Toward the end of May, Gardner had his *S. haemolyticus* at just the right strength.

The table of results of a scientific experiment often makes for dull reading. Occasionally, however, those results are so dramatic that following how they play out has all the pleasure of a good novel. What was called the mouse protection trial to quantify penicillin's effectiveness in living tissue began in Florey's lab in the Dunn School on Saturday, May 25, 1940. That this took place on a Saturday was "an indication of the urgency [Florey] felt, since normally no one would dream of starting an experiment at a week-end," Heatley later wrote. The urgency was justified; the two-page record foretells a new era in medicine.

At eleven A.M. Florey and Kent injected eight white mice with the smallest dose of virulent streptococci—about 110 million organisms—known to kill a mouse of average weight and returned them to their twelve-inch-diameter circular glass cages covered with a perforated zinc screen. The bottom of each cage was sprinkled with sawdust mixed with some crumbled biscuit to eat. At noon, mice Nos. 1 and 2 were given an injection of 5 ml of penicillin solution. Mice Nos. 3 and 4 received injections of 10 ml. The other four were controls, and received none. Nos. 3 and 4 were given only the one injection, but at two-fifteen P.M. mice Nos. 1 and 2, slightly stupefied by ether to make handling them easier, were given another 5 ml dose. They would receive additional penicillin at four-fifteen, six-twenty, and ten P.M.

A deadly dose of streptococcus is not immediately fatal, so for the first several hours after the initial injections, there was little to do but keep an eye on the mice in their cages and wait to see how the protected mice responded. Florey, Kent, and Heatley watched the animals throughout the afternoon. Around six P.M. Florey sent Kent home for the night. At six-twenty, mice Nos. 1 and 2 were given their next dose. By six-thirty, seven and one half hours after being injected with the streptococci, there was a clear trend. Mice Nos. 1 and 2 appeared to be very well. Mouse No. 3, Florey noted in the observation log, was "quite lively, cleaning itself and eating biscuit. Other not so lively." Mice Nos. 5 to 8 all "look quite sick. No attempt to eat. Eyes permanently closed. Heads drooped. Fur roughed. Breathing laboured."

Before seven P.M. Florey went home for dinner. Heatley had a bite to eat at a nearby snack bar and was heading back to the lab when he bumped into a friend, who persuaded him to come to a local pub for a meal, which they accompanied with a bottle of Mouton-Rothschild 1936, then an affordable pleasure.

Florey returned to give mice Nos. 1 and 2 their ten P.M. injection and immediately saw how marked was the difference among the mice. One of the controls, he noted, was "nearly dead. Others in a poor way." The two who had received just the single dose of penicillin were "in good condition, especially one," while mice Nos. 1 and 2 were "cleaning themselves and eating." However critical the experiment, Florey was not inclined to watch every moment to see how it unfurled. So far, the predicted result seemed in sight. After injecting the mice, he went home for the night. Heatley was back before eleven and would stay until the last of the controls died.

"As the events unfolded," Heatley said years later, "I saw what I was expecting." Just before midnight he wrote in the lab notebook that all four mice with penicillin were apparently well, but the controls were certainly not. "One mouse got up and staggered about for a few seconds, then fell down, twitched once or twice and was dead. Others very seedy." Heatley made a cross sign in red ink to mark the death. By one-thirty A.M. on May 26, the four protected mice had napped and awoken, but two more controls had died, noted by two more red crosses. At three twenty-eight A.M., Heatley noted that the last control "moved about drunkenly. With each inspiration lifted its head and opened its mouth widely. Respiration became slower, animal twitched and died."

One of the mice that received a single shot lived two days, the other six. Of those that received five shots, one lived thirteen days, the other indefinitely. What no one realized at the time is how little penicillin it actually took to save the mice that received it. Because of its effectiveness in earlier tests and the results of this one, Florey and the others assumed that their penicillin was quite pure. Before long, they would discover that in fact the mice had been given a drug that contained less than one half of 1 percent penicillin and more than 99 percent extraneous matter. Luck favored the ignorant. Had any of these impurities been particularly toxic, Florey later wrote, "the non-toxicity of penicillin might have been completely masked, with unpredictable results on subsequent work."

But this was unknown that night. Even at less than 1 percent purity, penicillin's spectacular abilities were abundantly evident. Heatley made a final red cross, and at three forty-five A.M. he closed up the lab without removing the dead but highly toxic mice from their cage; the night was too far gone to take all the necessary precautionary steps to dispose of them safely. Yet however late the hour and however expected the outcome of the experiment, the result was so clear and its implications so breathtaking that Heatley was overcome with "relief, joy, happiness." He got on his bicycle and began his ride home, the first light of day already in the sky. He had not gone far before the quiet was cut by an angry, "Halt! Who goes there?" and an aged Home Guardsman with a rifle stopped him. Heatley explained that he had been working at the Dunn School and was allowed to continue on. He made no mention that he had just witnessed the world change.

At eleven A.M. on Sunday, May 26, Florey, Chain, and Heatley returned to the lab for a prearranged meeting. All three recognized the importance of the unambiguous result, and each acknowledged the news pretty much according to character: Heatley said little, Chain was excited, and Florey, for whom understatement was a hallmark, reportedly said, "It looks quite promising," though even he could not maintain so sober a manner for long. When he called Margaret Jennings to tell her the news, he exclaimed, "It looks like a miracle." Then he set the course to make sure it was no miracle or fluke but a scientific fact. He wanted to test penicillin in groups of up to fifty mice, and he asked Heatley if he could double his production of mold broth, to two hundred liters a week.

That same morning the war in Europe took a severe downturn for the Allies, and it looked as though a miracle of another sort would be needed to rescue hundreds of thousands of British, French, and Belgian soldiers, trapped in northern France along the coast by Dunkirk, who had been routed by forces led by the then unknown General Erwin Rommel. At first, the British Admiralty thought they could rescue no more than forty-five thousand of them. Evacuation by the Royal Navy began the morning of May 26. When on May 27 bombing by the Luftwaffe made the harbor of Dunkirk unusable, it looked as if even fewer would be rescued. But then as Churchill wrote, "Life boats from liners in the London docks, tugs from the Thames, yachts, fishing craft, lighters, barges and pleasure boats . . . were called into service. By the night of the 27th a great tide of small vessels began to flow towards the sea, first to our Channel ports and thence [fifty-five miles] to the beaches of Dunkirk and the beloved Army." By June 4, this ragged flotilla had brought 350,000 men from Dunkirk to safety. But another million less fortunate troops in France were taken prisoner. Even the miracle of Dunkirk could not obscure how desperate the outlook was for Britain.

The same-day juxtaposition of the bright promise for humankind that penicillin offered and the bleak threat to civilization by the ever-advancing Nazis was a coincidence known at the time by only a half-dozen people in Oxford. That summer the Battle of Britain would test the country almost to its limit. An invasion of England appeared inevitable. In the House of Commons the next week, Churchill, who had been prime minister for less than a month, delivered his most celebrated speech: "We shall not flag or fail. . . . We shall defend our island, whatever the cost may be. We shall fight on the beaches, we shall fight on the landing grounds, we shall fight in the fields and in the streets, we shall fight in the hills. We shall never surrender." Brave words indeed from the leader of a virtually defenseless country whose only protection was the English Channel and Royal Navy, a gritty but outnumbered army and air force, and Home Guardsmen suspicious of scientists on bicycles in the middle of the night.

During the first two days of the evacuation of Dunkirk, former prime minister Neville Chamberlain and Lord Halifax, a member of Churchill's War Cabinet, advocated that Britain strike an agreement with Hitler to cut its losses against what looked like inevitable defeat. Even Churchill gave thought to the proposal, but when, on the evening of May 28, it was evident that a complete evacuation was possible, he told the War Cabinet that "nations which went down fighting rose again, but those who surrendered peacefully were finished." He was even more dramatic a few minutes later when he spoke to the whole cabinet: "If this long island story of ours is to end at last, let it end only when each of us lies choking in his own blood upon the ground." He received a standing ovation.

———

On May 27 and again on May 28, mouse protection experiments on ten and then sixteen animals were carried out. The amounts of strep-tococci and penicillin that were given varied, and these experiments made it evident that life or death was determined by the amount of penicillin maintained in the body. The ideal concentration could be found only by experiments that required far more penicillin than could then be made in the containers at hand.

June and July were months of intense work for Florey and his group, who at first kept the news of the early results of penicillin strictly to themselves. Florey didn't mention it even to John Fulton, his friend from his Rhodes scholar days and now Sterling Professor of Physiology at Yale University. Nor was he much more forthcoming in a June 11 letter to Mellanby: "As I told you recently, we have been working with a substance that gives the greatest promise of being an important chemotherapeutic substance." Without naming this sub-stance he talked about its strength even when highly diluted as well as its lack of toxicity, and then cautioned, "Naturally we do not wish anything to be said about this at the present stage." What Florey did wish for was to increase the size of the penicillin team and further solidify its financial backing.

Two weeks later there was a reply approving an increase in Chain's expenses, more money for Margaret Jennings to work full-time on penicillin, salaries for Duncan Gardner and Jean Orr-Ewing to work on the bacterial side, and for Edward Abraham to do "chemical work on the chemotherapeutic substance." Abraham and Chain now devoted all their time to researching penicillin's chemical composition so that they might purify the active substance.

Florey set the group to finding what was the minimum dose needed, and how often it needed to be given, to overcome various deadly bac-teria. Over a period of two days and nights at the start of July, Florey and Kent gave fifty mice triple the dose of streptococci given the eight in May; twenty-five of them received injections of penicillin every three hours, the rest none.

In a fluid motion, Kent would take a mouse by the tail, swing it onto the arm of his lab coat, grasp it by the back of the neck, turn it onto its back for the injection, then drop it back in the cage. Florey and Kent would go home for dinner and return about seven P.M. for the night. Kent picked out any of the mice that had died while Florey made a note. Florey grabbed what sleep he could in the bed that folded out of one wall in his office, while Kent managed on a camp cot.

The results of the experiment were as stunning as the first mouse trial. All the mice given no penicillin were dead within sixteen hours. Twenty-four of the treated mice were alive and still fine ten days later. An autopsy on the one protected mouse that died showed the cause of death to be an undetected and long-standing fatal internal disease.

While Florey and Kent kept a vigil in the lab, Gardner and the others returned home to sleep, but in the morning they rushed excitedly down to the laboratory to see the result of the night's work. The evidence defied even Gardner's usual understatement: "There could be no further doubt that penicillin was the very thing that doctors for a century had hoped and longed for."

As the war continued ever worse for Britain, these experiments were followed by others using different deadly organisms on groups of as many as seventy-five mice. Each experiment added to the plain evidence that in mice, anyway, penicillin was astonishingly potent. Florey was quick to point out that penicillin still had to be proved in a human, who is three thousand times the weight of a mouse.

For all of Florey's attention and the resources of the Dunn School that were poured into penicillin, it is important to note that it was far from the only work being done at the time. In July alone, Florey and his collaborators submitted to various journals two papers on lymphocytes, one on the mechanism of capillary contraction, and one on the effects of the removal of lymphoid tissue from the body.

In May, George Glister, a technical assistant who would eventually take over growing the mold, had joined the Dunn staff, much to Heatley's pleasure. After the first mouse protection trial, the two continued to tackle the problem of producing greater quantities of penicillin. Because of shortages caused by the war, there was no hope of simply ordering growing dishes, and, anyway, no one was yet certain what was the most effective vessel in which to grow it. As only a very shallow layer of medium was necessary, short, flat containers wasted less space than tall, round ones in the incubators and autoclaves. But finding an adequate quantity of anything remotely suitable for growing the mold was difficult.

In early June, Heatley tried to collect biscuit tins for growing the mold from various grocers in Oxford. He found a few but not enough, so Florey suggested he try in Reading, about halfway to London. Huntley and Palmers, a large biscuit company, did not have any square tins, but they gave Heatley a hundred big round ones. Huntley, Bourne and Stevens, a tin box manufacturer, gave him another dozen.

Tins were not the only makeshift equipment. The mail on June 13 brought Heatley a letter from his parents with a fragment of parachute silk, which he turned into two filtration bags on his landlady's sewing machine.

Heatley's diary entries during June and July give a good sense of life in the lab at this time, and of how his work on the extraction apparatus progressed:

June 15: "I went to register for National Service after lunch, then worked in the lab until 7 o'clock. Collected a pass from the military authorities in the Old Clarendon, for our lab is to be guarded by the Army after 7.0 p.m."

June 27: "George and I collected about 40 litres of P solution, and filtered it. In the afternoon tried the dustbin still I had designed, and it worked perfectly, although the cooling condenser was not quite efficient enough."

July 7: "Spent the evening making masks of silk, for handling the cultures in a sterile way."

July 8: "Tried out the first complete apparatus for extraction of P, but it did not seem to work well at all. Began to scheme out a new idea for suspending wicks or thread in ether, and running aqueous solution down them."

July 9: "Spent all day making a new P extractor, on the wick principle. Seemed to work fairly well, but the wicks soon became clogged with mess from the P."

July 17: "The whole of one batch of 30 tins was infected, so we discarded it. Set up a new batch of tins. Began to make a new P extracting device. The Professor showed me how to inject mice—he will be away tomorrow and wants me to do it for him then."

July 25: "Spent all day playing with the P-extracting apparatus. Gained several useful experiences, and I think it will work quite well eventually."

As the summer progressed, Heatley added more and more found objects to his collection of growing dishes—pie tins, trays, china plates; bed pans with a hollow handle/spout and removable lid, which were provided by the Radcliffe Infirmary, proved particularly useful; there were cracker tins and gas cans, lacquered to prevent destructive contact between penicillin and metal (until it was evident that autoclaving and chemical action peeled it away); there was even a dog bath.

All the while, the outlook for Britain's security grew dimmer. On June 22, General Philippe Pétain, the autocratic hero of the Battle of Verdun in World War I who had been brought into the government to help rescue the country in the current crisis, instead surrendered France to the Nazis and became head of the Vichy government.

"The Battle of France is over," Churchill said, "I expect the Battle of Britain is about to begin."

On July 10, it did, with Nazi bombing attacks on convoys of freighters in the English Channel bringing food and raw materials. Over the next four months the battle was fought in the sky as the Royal Air Force met wave after wave of fighters trying to destroy RAF fields. A safe outcome was not at all assured; rather, an invasion seemed all the more likely that summer.

If indeed there was an invasion, all British scientists whose research could help the Nazis knew that they would have to destroy their work so that it would not fall into the hands of the enemy. Destroying the work on penicillin meant there loomed the prospect of the Oxford group losing all they had accomplished because the only way to carry on the research was with the particular strain of *Penicillium notatum*. If the work was destroyed to avoid its secrets being captured, how could those who managed to get to safety resume the experiments?

Heatley came up with the answer. He suggested that if they rubbed spores of the mold into the fabric of their coats, the dingy brown motes would blend into the material and could lie dormant for years.

It was the reverse of the soldiers in World War I whose uniforms carried invisible bacteria and ready infection. The spores in *these* clothes could lead to a cure for all those ills. None of the group had a large wardrobe. With the spores safely tucked into the weave of their clothing, if they had to flee, Florey, Heatley, Chain, Gardner, and Jennings could carry their work out with them on their backs.

On September 7, the blitz of London and other major cities began and continued for fifty-seven consecutive nights; between September 7 and October 5, 50 million pounds of bombs were dropped on London; hundreds of thousands of Londoners spent the nights on the platforms and stairs of London Underground stations and in other shelters. By the time the bombing ended on October 31 and a stymied Hitler turned his attention to Russia, forty thousand Britons had been killed, another fifty thousand seriously wounded. The RAF had lost 832 fighters, the Luftwaffe 668 as well as 600 bombers. There was no invasion. "Never in the field of human conflict was so much owed by so many to so few," Churchill memorably told the nation.

Oxford was spared in the bombing: there was not a single air raid. So was Heidelberg. A long-held but unsubstantiated theory is that there was a secret agreement not to destroy the great universities. More likely is that Oxford was far inland and without major manufacturing plants. The war did not go as well for Fleming, whose house in London's Chelsea was bombed in March 1941. He was not injured.

Beyond the stress of the war and the heightened pace of the work on penicillin, the summer of 1940 was also a period of intense personal turmoil for Howard and Ethel. Though their marriage had been unsatisfactory for years, divorce was social suicide. For the sake of their children, they maintained an uneasy truce at home until Ethel's death in October 1966. Their false facade was painfully evident to anyone who knew them.

"I'm afraid your parents leave a great deal to be desired," Howard wrote in March 1966 to Charles, who was about to be married in New Haven, Connecticut, to his fiancée Sue Hopkins. "All I can say, looking back, is that I'd willingly exchange a really happy marriage for scientific distinction. I hope yours will go alright." Howard and Ethel, each as stubborn as the other, had long ago reached a point of mutual exasperation. Ethel, though she had severe heart problems and her doctors were adamant that she should not travel, was determined to be at the wedding. Howard then canceled his own plans to attend, even though he would be in the country to give a lecture in Texas. He continued:

> I do not know of any arrangements Ma has made and I do not intend to ask. She will be left entirely to look after herself.
>
> I think I need a session on the couch. What the lecture for Houston will be like God knows.
>
> All the best to both of you,
Dad

It may not be a surprise that Florey found succor with someone else. Margaret Jennings, who had become his assistant in October 1936, was necessarily a steady companion at work. She also provided a counterpoint to Ethel. She was physically healthy where Ethel suffered from deafness and other infirmities; a companion in his work without ever challenging him intellectually; and docile where Ethel was ambitious. In April 1968, two months after Florey's death, Margaret handwrote a note that was sealed in Florey's papers at the Royal Society, not to be opened until after her own death, which was in 1994.

> Howard had a tenderly romantic attitude towards women which was completely stultified in his relations with his first wife. . . . When he made me his mistress in 1940 his tender solicitude and wish to give me happiness through his physical powers, as well as by caring for me, were most touching. I was then separated from the husband who . . .

had done nothing to repair my physical and emotional immaturity. Howard understood this, and with great compassion, expressed particularly through his physical care and restraint, did all he could to help me. And I think I made him happy. I was his dream, and I always received with melting warmth his tributes; whether presents, or love making, or confidences which he was much too reserved to give elsewhere.

Of course I had anxieties and fears, particularly when we were exposed to the world, as going to the theatre, or traveling, but while he reasonably helped me and loved to care for me, and dominated me so far as to push me through the emotional barriers into doing the things that he had planned, he did not take charge and act the father-figure except when my fears made this necessary, and then he did it with reluctance. He stood independent, and, so far as I could accept this, he stood aside and expected me to have initiative and independence too. . . .

It is an interesting document in many ways, not least in that it offers her rationale for why she was willing to be a mistress for over twenty-five years. But it is the only side of the story that is recorded by any of the three principals.

Henry Harris, who followed Florey as Professor of Pathology at the Dunn School and was appointed Regius Professor of Medicine by Queen Elizabeth II, knew Margaret Jennings and both Floreys well. Harris's pioneering work on cell fusion led to, among other things, the development of monoclonal antibodies and his own discovery of tumor-suppressing genes. Now retired but still scientifically active, his unsentimental evaluations of all three are insightful and telling, and quite likely the best to be had from anyone who knew them all. While declarative in his views, Harris warns, "This is my surmise and my own reaction to these two women. There is very little in the way of fact."

Margaret and Ethel, he points out, were each difficult in their own way:

Margaret was the Honorable—the child of a 19th century plutocrat turned aristocrat. When Florey got started at Oxford, he wrote to Robert Webb at the Royal Free Hospital in London and asked for a slave to do routine work. Jennings was sent. She was married at the time but the union came apart, so the story goes, when she found her husband in bed with a nurse. She then set her cap on Florey. It shouldn't have taken Margaret long to land him. He was a fairly unhappy man. Ethel and Howard fought quite a bit and sexually they didn't go very well. Plus, as Florey once said to me, she was deaf as a post.

Although solicitous of Florey, "Margaret was a snobbish woman of rather modest ability. She used to speak to technicians in a way that today would precipitate a riot. Yet she was not a woman of any intellectual power but rather a woman who capitalized on her recent aristocratic background. Her one great talent was to turn Florey's papers into better prose."

Ethel, on the other hand, was not much of a stylist. "Florey called me in once and said, 'Harris, my wife is preparing to write a book on [the clinical application of] antibiotics. Can you turn it into English?'" Despite this drawback, Ethel had definite views on exactly how a sentence should be written. When she and Norman Heatley collaborated on a paper, he recalls having to "fight with her over every comma."

While Margaret had Florey's affection, apparently his was all she commanded at the Dunn School. Apart from her condescending manner, Harris says that "she tattled to Florey on what was going on in the lab; nobody in the lab could stand her. If Florey had become involved with Bardot, everyone would have thrown their caps in the air. For myself, I'd rather go to bed with a crocodile."

Margaret's reference in her archival note to her fear of being exposed while traveling refers in part to an incident in the early 1940s. Once their affair began, she and Florey would leave for vacations separately and at slightly different times (Florey often traveled without Ethel and the children) but then meet up in a place away from people they knew. At least that was the plan. On one of these trips, however, a friend of Duncan Gardner saw them on the beach in Normandy, although it is not clear if Ethel was told. The encounter was never mentioned among the three, and Ethel, Howard, and Margaret continued to play their parts in the charade. "It puzzled me," Gardner later wrote, reflecting the opinion of many in the lab, "that his sexual urges seemed to drive him away from his attractive wife, Ethel, to a very (to me) unattractive Margaret Jennings." Margaret accompanied Florey to Royal Society events and scientific meetings, ostensibly because they worked together on projects, and because of Ethel's deafness. For decades their liaison was one of the worst-kept secrets in Oxford and the subject of gossip around the workbench, yet no one who knew the story would speak of it outside the lab. The reason, Harris says, is simple.

"Florey dominated all his team. It was piety to the dead Florey not to say anything about Margaret. And I don't want to denigrate the man on account of his liaisons—look at the mistresses of Mahler, Kafka, and Einstein; these were very funny girls."

The difficulties Ethel coped with, both physical and emotional, weighed on her, Harris says. "Ethel once said to me, 'Life's hell, don't you agree?' I don't think she was a kindly person but she was decent and hospitable." He adds that his "impressions of the two women are common knowledge. The Florey marriage was dry and not very successful." As for Margaret, "Florey became involved with a schemer who then stayed with him legally; he made an honest woman of her. It's such a platitudinous story. He was not sexually adventurous but she was there and working late." Even so, it was a love affair that would sustain Florey until his death.

The damage from the Nazi bombings of Britain was so severe that many parents in large cities sent their children to live with relatives or even strangers in the country, less in harm's way. In July 1940, the immediate threat of a Nazi invasion and occupation led a group at Yale University to organize the evacuation of children from Oxford to the United States. Families in New Haven and other Eastern college cities opened their homes to care for these children for however long would be necessary and the parents of more than 125, aged one month to their teens, accepted this offer of sanctuary. Ethel and Howard Florey were among them.

The decision to send Paquita, ten, and Charles, five, to safety obviously brought out the same mixed emotions in the Floreys that it did in the parents of other children who were sent abroad. They had the trauma of deciding whether it was best for their children to remain in

Oxford amid the uncertainty of war or to travel across an ocean for an undetermined time. If travel was the choice, then there would be a separation of unknown length. There was as well the knowledge that Nazi submarines and U-boats were on the constant hunt for Allied sea traffic; through the beginning of July 1941, they sank over six hundred ships. Other concerns were part of the decision. Was it fair for some people to go to safety while others were left in danger? Ethel might have gone along on the trip as one of the mothers who accompanied the children, but because of her sense of community and her desire to be involved with what was clearly work of the highest importance, nothing could convince her to leave.

The trip was planned in secret, and Paquita and Charles had little forewarning that they would go to the United States; Charles was told he was going the day he left, or perhaps the day before; for some time he had heard whispering in the house and been admonished "not to 'tell anybody,'" but he "didn't know what we weren't to tell anybody." After Paquita was told the two of them might be sent abroad, she was kept home from school to avoid her inadvertently saying something to schoolmates about the trip. She came to feel that the secrecy of the plans and the lack of a firm date of departure "may be the reason I thought [my parents] wanted to get rid of me." The decision to send the children saddened Ethel more than Charles or Paquita could have imagined at the time. A friend of Ethel's told Paquita some years later that her mother was never the same after she and Charles left.

When the day of departure did come, Ethel and Howard accompanied their children by train to the docks of Liverpool and took their leave in two distinct ways.

"Dad didn't like fuss or emotional bother," Paquita told Gwyn Macfarlane nearly forty years after the event. "He just kissed us good-bye and told us to be good, but mother was terribly cut up and cried because she felt it was a dreadful thing for us to go alone." Howard and Ethel remained on the pier while she and Charles cried and waved as the ship pulled out.

When the list of children coming to America reached New Haven, John Fulton was elated to see the Florey children on it and immediately sent a cable to Howard.

OXFORD SAILING LIST JUST RECEIVED MAY WE CLAIM CHARLES AND PAQUITA
FOR DURATION

The response came three days later:

VERY MANY THANKS EXTREMELY KIND OF YOU

Fulton's work at Oxford and after had made him a prominent figure in medicine. His work in the 1920s and 1930s outlined basic con-
cepts of the working of the brain, and under his direction much
research on frontal lobotomy was conducted at Yale. His textbook
The Physiology of the Nervous System was in wide use in medical
schools throughout the world. His wife Lucia's family had made their
fortune in the China clipper trade. (Fulton's "in-laws are rotten with
coin," Florey wrote to Ethel in 1925.) The Fultons' large home in
Hamden, near New Haven, was atypical for a college professor, but
it had plenty of room for children, and it contained many reminders
of Oxford; Ackerman prints of the university hung on the walls of
Charles's bedroom.

The children's trip across the Atlantic included an unsuccessful submarine attack, which made it a routine one for a time in which ships
often were sunk. They arrived safely in Canada on July 21, though
not without confusion. The Cunard Line misidentified the ship and
sent an urgent message to Fulton and the Yale committee to come
immediately to Montreal. Once there, they were told there had been
a mistake and in fact there was no report of a boatload of children.
Eventually they all made it to New Haven, where Paquita caught the
attention of a reporter for the *New Haven Journal and Courier*:

"Paquita Florey, 10, traveled to New Haven with her five-year-old
brother, their mother and father remaining in England. En route to
the Community Center, with great delight she read a comic book she
had purchased in Montreal while Charles amused himself by pulling
on the bell cord of the bus. Asked if she liked the comic book, Paquita
said, 'Oh, yes, you see mother and father never allow me to read them
at home.' "

Fulton sent a cable to Florey, assuring him that

PAQ EG FLOURISHING

Florey immediately wrote to his friends, thanking them and at the same time releasing them of any obligation if the children should prove difficult:

My Dear John and Lucia,

We, as you can well imagine, are deeply grateful to you for so generously looking after our children. I hope you won't have too much cause to regret the sudden increase of your family. Your cable came today and we can sleep better—one rather gets the idea that there's a submarine every mile or two—but anyway that's over. I hope you will like the children—the girl is a willful creature at times and apt to be moody. They have few inhibitions and you'll probably soon find yourselves being called "Silly old John and Lucia" or something to that effect. The boy is a funny little chap, very interested in all that goes on and we have little doubt he will accommodate himself to any new surroundings—he left here in high spirits. I do hope you won't spoil them—be quite firm and don't let them pester you in any way. If you find them too much of a nuisance—they quarrel from time to time etc—just get rid of them to someone else—we will quite understand.

Life is beginning to change here now. There are plenty of aeroplanes about—all ours I think! They fly over the lab nearly all day and sometimes one can't hear oneself speak. All to the good. . . .

Work goes on in the lab though we are changing from the things we were working on to things of more practical importance. We are all very busy now as we think we have an entirely new line in chemotherapy, which will deal with gas gangrene among other things. There are lots of people working on wound healing and things of that sort and my impression is that medicine may get a big kick out of the war— as it did from the last one. . . .

Yours ever, H. W. Florey

Fulton was not worried about how the children would behave but rather, he wrote to Florey, how he and Lucia would be able to deal with them. A childless couple with an active intellectual and social life, they were about to dive into the turbulent waters of parenthood and were happy for the opportunity.

The first report on the children must have pleased the Floreys. In early August Fulton wrote:

> Paquita is a great credit to yours and Ethel's careful upbringing, most polite and with an unusually well developed social sense for a youngster of ten years. She works hard on Eg, telling him what to do and what not, all of which Eg takes very serenely, evidently reserving judgment whenever he receives a sisterly reprimand for having eaten his ice cream too fast or whatnot. . . . Lucia is at the moment a rather stern disciplinarian, so I think Ethel need not worry about their being spoiled. I am much more likely to spoil them than she is. They seem to have discovered that, although they still have moments of being a little terrified of me—at least Paquita does. Eg is terrified of no one, in fact I think he would walk up and shake hands with the Holy Ghost and ask after his health. He is so completely unspoiled in all his outgoingness and I hope nothing will happen to alter his spontaneity in any way.

Referring to the Battle of Britain and his support for American intervention in the war in Europe despite the opposition of isolationists, Fulton continued:

> You will be much in our thoughts these next weeks, my dear Howard, and I can only wish that we were a little nearer at hand to help more substantially in all that you are doing. . . . But we have our Lindberghs as you have your Mosleys, and I can only hope that we will succeed in suppressing them before it is too late. Meanwhile our affectionate greetings to you both.

Charles quickly adapted to America and life with the Fultons, but it was not so easy for Paquita. Studies of the deleterious effects of the separation of children from their mothers had yet to be done, although it required no psychological study to see how affected she was. Everything about her temporary home was different from her real one. The Fultons not only had no children, Paquita felt they also had "a lifestyle that excluded them, although their many material possessions helped make up for it."

What they clearly did have was a lifestyle that suited broad-minded adults. The Fultons were very well connected to many strata of society. Friends and acquaintances ranged from their neighbor the playwright Thornton Wilder (*Our Town* was a recent hit and *The Skin of Our Teeth* was about to be produced) to virtually every scientist or scientific official of high rank in America and Europe. One day their large home might be a reception for a group of biologists; on others there were what Paquita recalls as "arty parties with Thornton Wilder and some of his Bohemian friends. Uncle John was greatly admired, at least by certain women," and Lucia had an admirer or two herself. Drinks were never absent at Mill Rock nor was nude swimming frowned upon. Otherwise sedate New Haven women were known to disrobe and dance Isadora Duncan–style in the garden fountain.

John Fulton was an often-distant figure, but Paquita found he could also be "teasing and rather jolly." As he wrote to Howard, he was the counterpoint to Lucia's "stern disciplinarian." He did, however, have distinct ideas on how children should learn. Whenever Charles or Paquita would ask a question, he would tell them to look up the answer in one of the two sets of the *Encyclopedia Britannica* close at hand. While this might have been an effective learning technique if followed, the net effect was that the two children stopped expressing their curiosity. In an otherwise avuncular letter in response to Charles sent from camp one summer, he chided him for not identifying more birds. Still, Fulton was a staunch defender of Paquita and especially of Charles, whom Florey quite wrongly never felt measured up intellectually. "You have never thought he knew much," Fulton told Florey in 1956, when to Florey's amazement Charles was proving himself an excellent medical student, "but we have always felt that he knew much more than you realized."

Despite the turmoil in Florey's personal life, at Oxford work pressed on with increasing urgency.

8

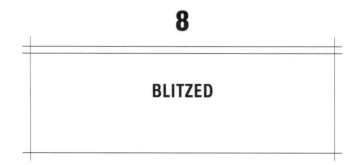

BLITZED

At the time Paquita and Charles left for the United States, it was clear to Florey that the Dunn School group could not produce penicillin on a scale large enough to supply all that was required for additional trials, and he hoped he could enlist the help of a drug company. At the suggestion of Sir Henry Dale, the president of the Royal Society, in mid-July two leading scientists from the Wellcome Laboratories came to Oxford to see penicillin firsthand, and later a few experiments were carried out at their plant. The timing, however, was terrible. Shortly after their visit, one of the worst periods of bombing began. Even without this added complication, Wellcome officials felt the company was at full capacity producing vaccines and antitoxins and doing other war work. Under these circumstances, penicillin did not seem to them important enough to commit extra resources.

There was by now an added incentive for the Oxford group to carry on, because regardless of others' doubts, they were convinced of penicillin's high potential. "The months spent in accumulating stocks and increasing the output, with all their disappointments and trials, are not likely to be forgotten by those involved," Florey later wrote. "The possibility that the drug might be of value in treating war injuries provided by this time a powerful stimulus to persevere."

A great leap forward in purifying penicillin was made in August when, at Edward Abraham's suggestion, the first attempt was made to separate crude penicillin in its ether solution through a process called chromatography. Chromatography separates materials and their pigments according to differences in how quickly they are absorbed by a powder that will not dissolve. The most absorbent bits of matter will collect and form a top layer; other components collect lower down, according to their absorbent properties, leaving several distinct bands of separated material.

After the penicillin filtrate was poured through a glass tube filled with alumina powder, four clearly colored bands were delineated. There was little penicillin in the top brownish-orange band. The second, pale yellow band was about 80 percent penicillin and free of contaminants that could cause a fever. The orange third layer had some penicillin and some or all of the fever-causing contaminants, and the bottom brownish or reddish-violet purple band had practically no penicillin but was instead full of impurities. Using a small spatula, the yellow band was lifted out, along with the powder just below and above it to capture smaller amounts of penicillin that might be in it. The powder was then washed four times over seven and a half hours in a neutral solution (neither acid nor alkali, called a buffer) to clear off the alumina. This process was then repeated a half-dozen times. The resulting fluid was deep reddish-orange that turned yellow when diluted and which had a faint smell and bitter taste.

All this was designed to produce a salt—a crystal—of penicillin so that the secret of the chemical structure of the active ingredient could be unlocked by X-rays shot through the crystal, exposing a pattern on film along with the address of every atom and molecule. It was not enough to have a powder that cured people. Growing mold and fishing penicillin out of broth was a necessary start, but it was critical to know its chemical nature so that it could be more efficiently produced.

Also during the latter months of 1940, Abraham and his colleagues showed for the first time that organisms could become resistant to penicillin. In the bacterial version of Friedrich Nietzsche's famous dictum, "What doesn't kill me makes me stronger," they showed that growing a strain of staphylococcus in ever-increasing concentrations of penicillin over a period of about four months increased resistance a thousandfold.

Two months after the first mouse protection trial, Florey was ready to announce the preliminary results of the work at Oxford. The August 24, 1940, issue of *The Lancet* carried a two-page article entitled "Penicillin as a Chemotherapeutic Agent," signed in alphabetical order by Chain, Florey, Gardner, Heatley, Jennings, Orr-Ewing, and Sanders. The article is sober in tone, understated in expression, and earthshaking in what it suggests, much like "Molecular Structure of Nucleic Acids," James D. Watson and Francis H. C. Crick's 1953 two-column paper in *Nature,* which introduced the double helix and disclosed the secret of DNA. Judging by these two papers, it seems almost axiomatic that the more important the discovery, the shorter the paper, and the drier the recitation of facts. Perhaps it is a defensive strategy to stake a claim to ensure credit but to avoid controversy.

The paper begins: "In recent years interest in chemotherapeutic effects has been almost exclusively focused on the sulphonamides and their derivatives. There are, however, other possibilities notably those connected with naturally occurring substances."

Rather like a minuet, with its prescribed forward balancing, bowing and toe pointing, the paper follows the protocol of politeness and exposition that envelops scientific publication, however pyrotechnic the results being reported. With necessary good manners, the earlier work of Fleming, Raistrick, and Reid is noted, followed by a slight jab pointing out the inability of these three to isolate penicillin. Details are given of the therapeutic experiments done using *Streptococcus pyogenes*, *Staphylococcus*, and *Clostridium septique,* including the amounts of bacteria and penicillin used and the numbers of mice that lived (those that received enough penicillin) and died (those that received little or none).

"The results are clear cut," the paper concludes, "and show that penicillin is active *in vivo* against at least three of the organisms inhibited *in vitro*. . . . Penicillin does not appear to be related to any chemotherapeutic substance in present use, and is particularly remarkable for its activity against the anaerobic organisms associated with gas gangrene." A footnote at the end thanked the Rockefeller Foundation, the MRC, and the Nuffield Trust for their financial support.

This news was as explosive as the prose is calm and flat. One of the most feared and deadly of war infections could be cured. The style is mirrored near the end of Watson and Crick's paper that unveils the secret of life: "It has not escaped our notice that the specific pairing we have postulated immediately suggests a possible copying mechanism for the genetic material."

On the other hand, what fanfare is needed when you're changing the course of medicine or unveiling the secrets of life?

The London Blitz commenced the day before the article appeared. Even with the immediacy of war, it was not a matter of vanity for Florey to think that the *Lancet* paper would be regarded as a signal achievement and that penicillin's promise would galvanize the interest of pharmaceutical companies. It was, however, in vain.

A note by the editors of the *Lancet* said of penicillin, "What its chemical nature is, and how it acts, and whether it can be prepared on a commercial scale, are problems to which the Oxford pathologists are doubtless addressing themselves." (The note seems to serve as something of a disclaimer by the editors that the chemical issue was not being neglected but in light of penicillin's possible importance, especially in wartime, they felt the paper should be published immediately.)

It is a good thing that the Oxford pathologists were appropriately addressing themselves, because no one else evinced any intention of doing so. The hopes Florey had that the *Lancet* article would arouse the interest of pharmaceutical companies—or even just one company— were for naught. It would be another nine months before one showed anything close to serious interest. Florey quickly realized that he and the others at Oxford were the only people who believed that penicillin could be tried before its chemistry was understood. However much more time it would add to the process, it was up to the team at the Dunn School to brew and extract the large amount of penicillin necessary to conduct tests on humans.

Even Fleming held the typical view at the time of penicillin's prospects: "Penicillin has not yet been tried in war surgery [for contaminated wounds] and it will not be tried until some chemist comes along and finds out what it is and if possible manufactures it."

"Fortunately," Florey added later, "this view, in the event, was not justified."

This view, however, was a logical long-term aim. If chemists could unravel the structure of penicillin, they might then be able to find a means of synthesizing it economically. This would make fermentation plants obsolete overnight, just as the advent of synthetic indigo in 1897 made obsolete the indigo plantations in India and elsewhere in the Far East. It was the drug companies' fear of just this possibility that dampened their interest in putting much money into penicillin at this stage.

Not only did the *Lancet* paper fail to capture the interest of the pharmaceutical companies, it caught the attention of very few scientists. Two of those who reacted were Edward Mellanby and Alexander Fleming. Neither of their responses could possibly have been what Florey expected.

On August 27, Mellanby wrote a letter to Florey that begins innocuously enough:

> I forwarded a copy of your letter concerning the possibility of sodium chloride lack in the army in the east to the War Office who reply that this has been thought of and every precaution taken to see that conditions like miner's cramp do not develop.

Mellanby then launches into what looks as if it will be a paean of congratulation but very soon becomes a reprimand and a grievance:

> I read your penicillin paper with great interest and it seems clear that you are on to a very good subject. I hope it develops as well clinically as it promises. I noted at the end of the paper that you gave a great boost to the Rockefeller Foundation for having supported this work and that the Medical Research Council had to play a very minor rôle. I doubt whether this is in accordance with the facts and, if you go out of your way to say that one member has got a Rockefeller fellowship, I think it is only reasonable that you should also mention the fact that several other members of the team were being supported by the Medical Research Council. The list would prove a striking one. I understand that the grants that are being held by individuals mentioned in the publication as part authors of this particular work are as follows:

FINANCIAL SUPPORT GIVEN BY
MEDICAL RESEARCH COUNCIL FOR PENICILLIN RESEARCH

	Personal	Expenses
Professor H. W. Florey	—	£50
Mrs. M.A. Jennings (part-time)	£200	—
Miss J. Orr-Ewing	200	350
E. Chain	300	100

I shall be surprised if the Rockefeller Foundation are supporting the work to anything like this extent. [He would soon be very surprised.]

It seems to me that your method of dealing with this matter is wrong tactics, partly because most of the grants that the Rockefeller Foundation give for medical research in this country follow discussion between O'Brien and me, and partly because, if you have a good thing in your own country, you might as well give it proper credit and not follow those people who, in cases of research, find it more convenient to give foreigners boosts than their own colleagues. Having said this, I salute you.

Everyone likes credit for backing a winner, especially a long shot, and Mellanby was worried that the MRC's bet had been obscured. His ire would grow when he learned that Florey had skirted the MRC for his 1939 Rockefeller grant, and he would feel triply stung. One of his stars was the recipient of a large grant, and no one at the MRC knew it. The grant had lessened Florey's reliance on the MRC and provided him some freedom, again without anyone at the MRC realizing it. And Florey had tweezered out this money soon after Mellanby had been unable to persuade the Rockefeller Foundation to help bridge the MRC's funding gap. Florey was unbowed by Mellanby's bluster and unimpressed by his accounting. On August 29, he replied:

Thank you for your letter—I am sorry to have troubled you about the salt.

I am also sorry for the annoyance the article has caused you but I hardly think "—financial assistance from the Rockefeller Foundation, the Medical Research Council and the Nuffield Trust—" suggests that a "great boost to the Rockefeller Foundation" has been given at the expense of the Medical Research Council.

As submitted to the *Lancet* the acknowledgements were as follows:

"In addition to the facilities provided by the University we have had financial assistance from the Rockefeller Foundation for technicians' salaries and expenses, from the Medical Research Council for expenses and personal grants to E. Chain, M. A. Jennings, and J. Orr-Ewing. The Nuffield Trust pays part of the salary of A. D. Gardner, and wages of his technician. To all of these we wish to express our thanks. N. G. Heatley has held a Rockefeller Fellowship."

They cut it down to that published. I am afraid it did not occur to me that the mention of Heatley (which they left in for some reason) would cause so much offence, so that I did not insist on having the full acknowledgements printed as submitted. This, in the event, was an error of judgment on my part.

The Rockefeller Grant has nothing to do with O'Brien whom I have never succeeded in interesting in the work here. I have dealt with the chemical side of the Foundation. They have always been sympathetic and most satisfactory to deal with: the negotiations with them started before I ever approached the Medical Research Council, but, owing to the difficulties of the war situation the European representative could not give me a positive statement as to what they would do till the end of 1939. In the end they gave 5,000 dollars (£1,200) for the year to be expended on good technicians, some expenses and capital expenditure for some expensive pieces of apparatus. Of this £1,200., £1,000. is being devoted to the penicillin work. This is in addition to Heatley's fellowship (£300. p.a.).

The figures you give do not apply solely to penicillin. . . . The correct figures for assistance from the Medical Research Council for penicillin work during the past year . . . at a maximum . . . amounts to £800. against about £1,300. from the Rockefeller people. You will thus see that there are very good reasons for thanking the Rockefeller Foundation for their generous assistance to the penicillin work.

I have always expressed my gratitude to you for Medical Research Council assistance, but, on the other hand, I am not aware of having

asked you to finance anything which did not produce the results anticipated.

Mellanby responded on September 3, still picking at nits but also
signaling a retreat, like a father who suddenly realizes he now has a
grown child to contend with.

I think you have given me a good but not a perfect answer to my
letter. . . .
   It was, of course, wrong of the Lancet people to alter your original
acknowledgements so as to give a distorted view of the situation but,
after all, you are responsible for the published statement. I give you full
credit for having the best intentions in this matter but not for carrying
them out. . . .
   When . . . you proceed to point out that only £800 of the total grant
of £2000 a year now being given to you by the Medical Research Council is being devoted to penicillin work, I feel you are engaged in special
pleading. However, the Lord be with you and, if you can get the penicillin to cure cases of human bacterial infection, I will forgive you a
good deal more than your misdeeds in the present instance.

In between the letters from Mellanby, Fleming arrived at the Dunn
School on September 2 after he telephoned Florey the evening before
to arrange the visit. It all transpired so quickly that many in the group
working on penicillin were surprised by his arrival, probably none
more than Chain, who thought Fleming was dead.

After Fleming abandoned penicillin in 1932, he turned much of his
attention to vaccines. In 1934, he coauthored the lengthy book *Recent
Advances in Serum and Vaccine Therapy*, and after sulfonamides
became available in 1936, he concentrated his experiments on them.
Between 1932 and 1940, he published fourteen scientific papers. In
the same period, Florey published over fifty.

When Heatley was told about the impending visit, he raised the
question of what, if anything, of the Oxford work should not be
shared with Fleming. Florey decided that he should be given any infor-

mation he wanted, and when Heatley described the growing of penicillin, he held back nothing in his two-hour presentation. Apart from telling Florey and Chain that he had come to see what the Oxford group had done "with my old penicillin," Fleming had little to say as he was shown the production and testing labs, though he did pay close attention to all he was shown and told. He returned to London with a small sample of the best penicillin but without leaving compliments for the work that had been done. Fleming tested the sample he had been given and was impressed by its potency; milligram for milligram, it was vastly stronger than any sulfa drug.

"It only remains for your chemical colleagues to purify the active principle, and then synthesize it," he wrote to Florey on November 15, "and the sulphonamides will be beaten." Which meant the decidedly mixed result for Fleming that medicine would be dramatically improved but also that his work for the past five years on sulfonamides essentially would be useless, because penicillin was better in so many respects. Fleming's future reputation now rested on receiving credit for his initial work that caught Chain's eye and led to the advance by the Dunn School group.

Unknown to Florey, there was someone besides Fleming and Mellanby who took a strong interest in the *Lancet* article. Dr. Martin Henry Dawson, a specialist in bacterial endocarditis at the Columbia University College of Physicians and Surgeons in New York, hoped that penicillin would save patients with this staphylococcal infection of the lining of the heart or its valves that infects the blood as well and was then a nearly uniformly fatal disease. (Streptococcus is the root of the subacute version of the disease.) Henry Dawson would come to understand better than most doctors the problems of doomed patients: in 1941, he was diagnosed with the degenerative neurological disease myasthenia gravis, which would kill him in April 1945. He left hope for finding a cure for his disease to specialists in that field and determined to do what he could for those afflicted with a malady whose course he might change.

In early September, Dawson wrote to Chain, asking for a sample of the Oxford mold. At the same time, he found a culture of Fleming's mold at the Pennsylvania Department of Agriculture and, along with Dr. Gladys Hobby, a microbiologist, and Dr. Karl Meyer, a biochemist, set up a penicillin production factory not dissimilar to the one at Oxford.

"Soon hundreds of two-liter flasks with *Penicillium notatum* growing on a modified Czapek-Dox medium lined every classroom laboratory bench at the Columbia University Medical School," Hobby later wrote. "We did not plan then to study fermentation processes for the production of penicillin. Rather we naively undertook 'to make some penicillin' " and to "establish that it would provide a therapeutic response." They had no incubators large enough for their work but soon discovered that the penicillin cultures could be grown in sanitary conditions in flasks incubated under the seats of a two-story amphitheater, at least for the eight or nine months that the temperature in the room was warm enough. The still for evaporating the solvents during the extraction of penicillin was set up on a fire escape to ensure safe venting.

Dawson and his colleagues quickly confirmed the Oxford results and, by October 15, had enough crude penicillin to inject two patients with small doses; these were the first humans to be given injections of the drug and receive what is known as systemic treatment. Unfortunately, there was not enough penicillin to improve the condition of the patients. Dawson delivered a paper on their findings at the May 1941 meeting of the American Society for Clinical Investigation. The *New York Times* ('GIANT' GERMICIDE YIELDED BY MOLD) and the *Philadelphia Evening Bulletin* (GERM KILLER FOUND IN COMMON MOLD) reported details of it. Although the paper was not published in a medical journal and these news reports did not arouse any general interest—Florey would not hear of this work for months—Dr. Wallace Herrell of the Mayo Clinic in Minnesota immediately started research into the drug.

A few American drug companies also began some preliminary research. Dr. Selman Waksman, a soil biologist at Rutgers University with a long-standing interest in antimicrobial substances and a consultant to nearby Merck and Company, convinced scientists there to look into penicillin. (Later Waksman would find four antibiotics, most notably streptomycin, which, unlike penicillin, was effective against TB. He won the Nobel Prize for physiology or medicine in 1952.) Also, Dr. Geoffrey Rake at E. R. Squibb and Sons began some experiments with penicillin, as did scientists at Charles Pfizer and Company (now Pfizer Inc.). By the fall of 1941, Pfizer was sending the Dawson group daily shipments of penicillin fermentation liquor to assay and use in their own research.

The work at Columbia was the most thorough in the United States to this time, but it was not the first. In 1933, Roger Reid, a graduate student at Pennsylvania State College, read Raistrick, Clutterbuck, and Lovell's 1932 paper. He decided to look into what he termed the "bacterial-inhibitory" qualities of *Penicillium notatum* and requested and received a sample of the culture from Fleming. Reid's professor supposedly dissuaded him from using penicillin as the subject of his doctoral thesis because the professor felt that penicillin was not an important enough topic. Reid did, however, confirm Raistrick, Clutterbuck, and Lovell's finding that penicillin was unstable, and, because like them he was unable to extract an active substance, he abandoned his work on it. Reid's failure did not deter a few scientists and at least one drug company—Eli Lilly and Company—from asking for a sample of the culture.

In 1936, the general superintendent at E. R. Squibb and Sons decided on the basis of the Raistrick paper to see whether penicillin merited thorough research. He assigned the Squibb librarian, herself an organic chemist, to survey all the literature and make a recommendation. She did and made a logical one based on the available facts: ". . . in view of the slow development, lack of stability and slowness of bacterial action shown by penicillin, its production and marketing as a bactericide does not appear practicable." Even so, some additional work was done there.

For the next several years interest in penicillin remained sporadic and isolated, and then it was threatened with becoming a sideshow altogether as American scientists turned their attention to other investigations. One exception was René Dubos, the French-American microbiologist and environmentalist who coined the injunction "Think globally, act locally." In 1939 he isolated tyrothricin from the soil bacteria *Bacillus brevis*. It was later shown to contain two separate antibiotics, gramicidin and tyrocidine, and some scientists thought that these might be more effective than penicillin until continued research demonstrated that while tyrothricin protected mice against many harmful bacteria and offered them significant protection against the progenitors of pneumonia, it had several toxic side effects when injected.

In January 1940, scientists at the New Jersey–based pharmaceutical company Merck and Company cultivated *P. notatum*, with the assumption that the study of penicillin would probably uncover other organisms with similar antibiotic properties, and three staff members were hired "to prepare useful chemicals by fermentation and to study isolation of therapeutic substances from micro-organisms." Not everyone thought this a useful idea. One executive later recalled "so-called experts urging Merck not to waste time on" penicillin, and, in fact, much of the year passed while interest in gramicidin flared up and then died. It was the fall of 1940 before Merck began to look for penicillin's active principle. Even then, American research into penicillin was still in its infancy.

A continually vexing problem for Heatley was finding enough appropriate vessels for growing the five hundred liters of penicillin filtrate a week now needed for further experiments. He fiddled around with a number of designs and eventually decided that the most efficient containers were the lidded bedpans he had been given by the Radcliffe Infirmary. Unfortunately, they were now using more modern, lidless versions, and there were no more of the old left, so he had to search for a firm that could cheaply make what he needed. The makers of Pyrex glassware were willing to help, but they wanted £500 (the equivalent buying power of about $25,000 in 2004) for the container mold alone, plus an additional amount for each item, an impossible price for the Dunn School budget. Anyway, the shortest delivery time they could offer was six months, hopelessly too long to wait.

Heatley then came up with the notion of having less-expensive slip-cast ceramic vessels made, and, on October 18, he drew sketches of possible shapes. He mailed them along with a note to a friend in Stoke-on-Trent in the Potteries District of Staffordshire, who, on October 29, sent a telegram saying that the firm of James Macintyre and Company might be of help.

On October 30, Heatley caught a delayed morning train to Stoke, about 120 miles northwest of Oxford, which was further delayed when it ran into an air raid just before Birmingham. At the pottery, the next morning, Heatley and a model maker came up with a square-sided design that looked like a cross between a rectangular hot-water bottle and an old-fashioned bedpan. It was about eleven inches long, nine inches wide and two and a half inches deep; its flat surface allowed for easy stacking. A sloped spout at one end was used for filling and emptying. The vessels were just the right size to hold a liter of broth 1.5 centimeters (.6 of an inch) deep. They were made of cheap impervious stoneware or porcelain that was glazed on the inside to allow for sterilization. (Not glazing the outside saved money and also made them less slippery to handle.) The price worked out to about ten shillings each—about $2.

The new vessels could not arrive soon enough to suit Florey. "Heatley has gone to Burslem today to see a pottery firm there to see what can be done," he wrote to Mellanby on October 31. "I am afraid the work is now almost completely held up because of the rusting of the tins we were brewing the stuff in."

The first samples arrived in Oxford on November 18 and, Heatley wrote in his diary, "were much admired." After tests were done to make sure they worked as anticipated, five hundred were ordered; later, another two hundred were made.

Throughout the fall of 1940, Heatley worked in a number of areas: he continued to modify his countercurrent extraction machine; his jack-of-all-trades ability drew the attention of some members of the Emergency Blood Transfusion Service, who visited the lab to learn his method of sharpening hypodermic needles; and, of course, he worked to double the output of penicillin. The war was never far away. One day while having tea with Edward Abraham, Abraham showed him

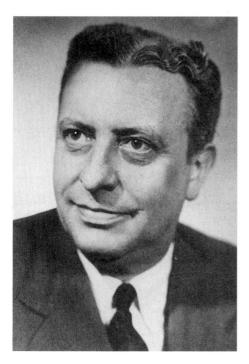

John Fulton met Howard Florey when they were Rhodes Scholars and was probably the reserved Florey's closest friend. An influential scientist at Yale and in American medicine, Fulton's support when Florey and Norman Heatley sought American help with penicillin in 1941 was invaluable.
COURTESY OF CHARLES FLOREY

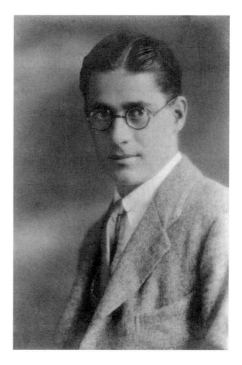

Howard Florey in the 1920s.
COURTESY OF CHARLES FLOREY

Howard Florey as a boy in Australia. His parents dressed him and kept his hair like this until he was eight.
COURTESY OF CHARLES FLOREY

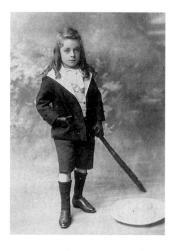

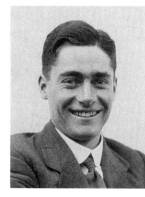

Howard Florey in the 1920s.
COURTESY OF CHARLES FLOREY

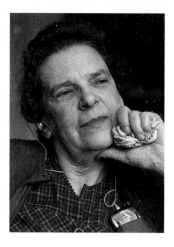

Ethel Florey, circa 1960. Her clinical trials of penicillin in the early 1940s at last enabled her to do meaningful medical work after she gave up her budding career as a doctor and left Australia to marry Howard in 1926.
COURTESY OF CHARLES FLOREY

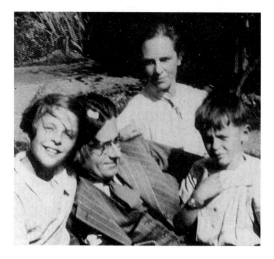

Howard and Ethel Florey with their children Paquita (*left*) and Charles, probably around the time the children were sent to the United States during World War II. COURTESY OF SIR WILLIAM DUNN SCHOOL OF PATHOLOGY

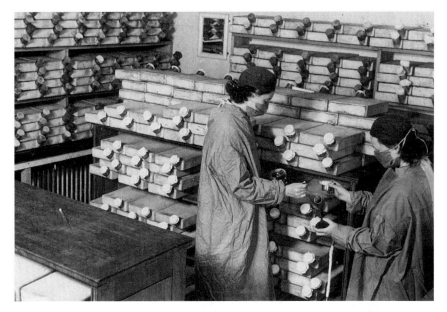

"Penicillin Girls" tending the Heatley-designed vessels for growing penicillin mold at the Sir William Dunn School in Oxford. COURTESY OF NORMAN HEATLEY

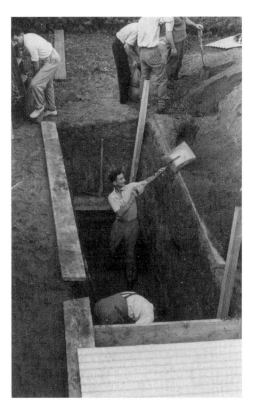

Norman Heatley (with shovel) and other Dunn School scientists digging an air-raid shelter behind the school, 1939. COURTESY OF NORMAN HEATLEY

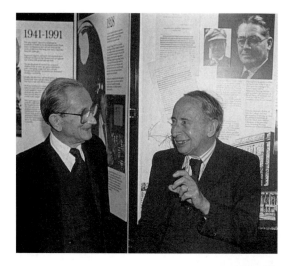

Norman Heatley (*left*) and Edward Abraham at an exhibit marking the fiftieth anniversary of the work on penicillin at Oxford. Florey's photograph is on the wall above Abraham. COURTESY OF NORMAN HEATLEY

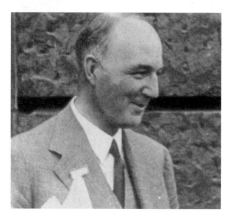

Edward Mellanby, the secretary of the Medical Research Council, controlled the purse strings for British scientific grants. His support for Florey influenced the choice of the Pathology Chair at Oxford in 1935, which paved the way for the development of penicillin. COURTESY OF CHARLES FLOREY

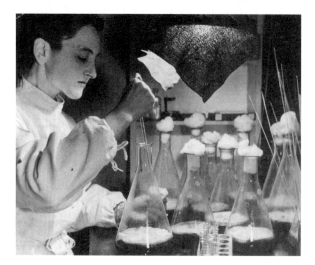

Margaret Jennings, Florey's inseparable assistant, taking a sample from a culture of penicillin mold. COURTESY OF CHARLES FLOREY

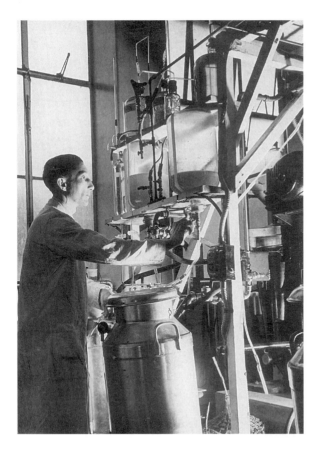

Gordon Sanders
tending to the
penicillin extraction
apparatus he designed.
COURTESY OF
NORMAN HEATLEY

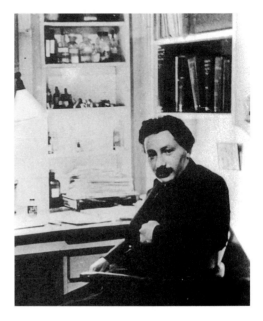

Ernst Chain at the Sir William
Dunn School, Oxford, looking
remarkably like Einstein.
COURTESY OF SIR WILLIAM DUNN
SCHOOL OF PATHOLOGY

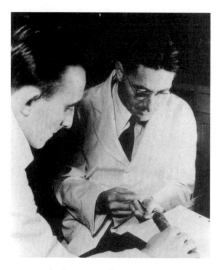

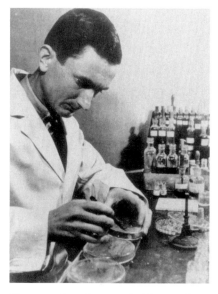

Howard Florey (*right*) and James Kent, Florey's animal technician for most of his career, injecting the tail vein of a mouse, probably with a very early penicillin preparation. COURTESY OF SIR WILLIAM DUNN SCHOOL OF PATHOLOGY

Norman Heatley, probably working on a penicillin assay, circa 1940. COURTESY OF SIR WILLIAM DUNN SCHOOL OF PATHOLOGY

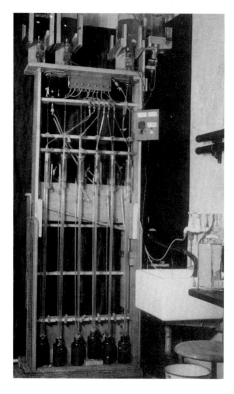

Norman Heatley's 1941 homemade countercurrent extraction apparatus for penicillin. The frame is made from a bookshelf discarded by the Bodleian Library; Heatley made most of the glass tubing and fashioned the copper coils and nozzles. The machine included colored lights and a doorbell. Total cost: about £5. COURTESY OF SIR WILLIAM DUNN SCHOOL OF PATHOLOGY

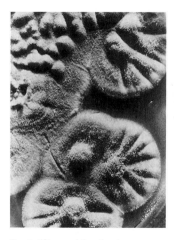

Penicillin mold colonies.
COURTESY OF SIR WILLIAM
DUNN SCHOOL OF PATHOLOGY

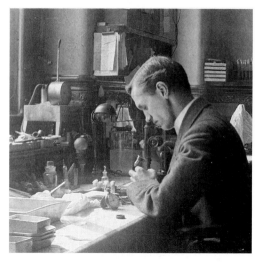

Alexander Fleming in his St. Mary's Hospital laboratory, circa 1909. He worked in this room for forty-nine years. COURTESY OF ALEXANDER FLEMING LABORATORY MUSEUM (ST. MARY'S NHS TRUST)

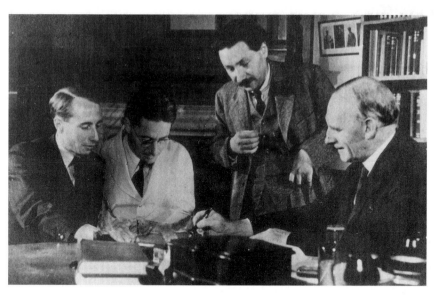

(*Left to right*) Edward Abraham, Howard Florey, Ernst Chain, and Robert Robinson discussing the chemical structure of penicillin, 1943. Abraham and Chain postulated that penicillin's structure was unique; Robertson, head of the Dyson Perrins Laboratory next door to the Dunn School and the 1947 Nobel laureate in chemistry, strongly disagreed. In 1945 X-ray crystallography determined that Abraham and Chain's solution was correct. Abraham went on to develop cephalosporin. COURTESY OF SIR WILLIAM DUNN SCHOOL OF PATHOLOGY

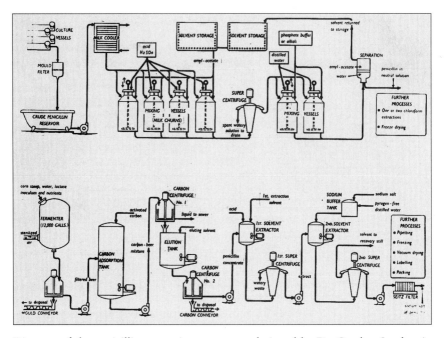

Diagram of the penicillin extraction apparatus designed by Dr. Gordon Sanders in late 1941, while Heatley was working on penicillin in America. For two years, the jury-rigged equipment at the Dunn School constituted the largest extraction plant in Britain. COURTESY OF SIR WILLIAM DUNN SCHOOL OF PATHOLOGY

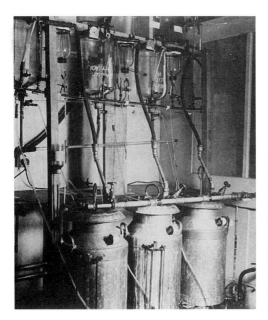

Milk churns used in the extraction of penicillin, December 1941. Sanders's device also employed a six-foot bathtub and used trash cans as steam-heated stills. The only pieces of true scientific equipment were two centrifuges. COURTESY OF SIR WILLIAM DUNN SCHOOL OF PATHOLOGY

the large pistol he had been given as one of the Home Guard, which he often kept tucked into his belt as he rode around Oxford on his motorcycle.

On December 22, 1940, Heatley borrowed the small Ford van assigned to Chain's blood service and drove to Stoke-on-Trent, where he spent the night. Early on December 23, the first 174 of the new ceramic culture vessels were loaded piece by piece and packed in straw, and Heatley drove through a snowstorm back to Oxford. The round-trip was made even more difficult because the roads of Britain were now unmarked, so that if the Nazis did invade, there would be no directional signs to help them get around the country.

Heatley and four helpers spent Christmas Eve making medium, filling the new vessels with a liter of mold broth, and sterilizing them. Then on Christmas Day he sowed seventy-six of the vessels with a spray gun.

On New Year's Eve he took stock of the past twelve months: "What a year! . . . The latter part of the year I have left research entirely, and have been concentrating on the production of P on a large scale. Now, with the help of George Glister, Ruth Callow, and Claire Inayat we are beginning to grow P nearly one thousand times the scale on which I was growing it a year ago."

Work at the lab continued at such a pace that Florey asked the MRC for money to pay trained research assistants; for a number of reasons, prominently that so many young men were going to war, none could be found. Instead, Florey turned to a group of young women with no scientific training who would play an indispensable part in the advancement of penicillin. Ruth Callow (now Parker), the sister of Chain's assistant Donald Callow, and Claire Inayat were the first of what became six Penicillin Girls. Ruth was seventeen when she started work in December, "a slip of a girl," Heatley wrote. She had hoped to be a children's nurse and had begun studies at Birmingham Hospital. Then she caught scarlet fever, and the air raids came, and the required three-year commitment was too daunting. She left after eight weeks and would have to wait until she was eighteen to go into ordinary nursing. After her brother told her about the job, she was interviewed by Heatley, who asked if she could tie knots—dexterity was essential for the work—and if she could lift a full four-liter bottle. She stayed eight years.

Soon Megan Lancaster (now Nurser) answered an ad in the *Oxford Times* and joined the group. She was sixteen and a half and went with her mother for the interview. Heatley immediately hired her. Like the others—Betty Cooke, Peggy Gardner, and Patricia McKegney—she worked from nine A.M. to six P.M. weekdays, nine A.M. to one P.M. Saturdays but stayed later if there was still work to be done, and occasionally went in on a Sunday. At lunch she usually biked two miles home to eat but sometimes went to a ration points–free "British restaurant" in the Oxford town hall, where diners were served two vegetables and meat in an enamel bowl "and pudding afterward, if we were lucky."

Under the immediate direction of George Glister, the Penicillin Girls washed and sterilized the ceramic vessels, filled them with medium, and spray-gunned the spores. Once they had done that, they wheeled them on a cart to what had been the students' preparation room, joined by a door to Heatley's lab, and which now was an incubator kept at 75.2 degrees Fahrenheit (24 degrees Celsius). Transporting the vessels could be noisy. "The wretched things rattled," Megan Nurser would say. Abraham and Chain's lab was beneath Heatley's, and the commotion sometimes disturbed their experiments.

After the penicillin mold had grown for several days, the girls suctioned off the fluid and recharged the pots. They wore surgical masks, caps, and gowns (changed each week) to fend off contamination of the broth, and they worked under conditions that no safety inspector today would allow; fumes of chloroform and ether and the pear scent of amyl acetate permeated the air. (The mold, however, had no particular odor.) They took ferrous sulfate to replenish the iron in their blood neutralized by the amyl acetate and had periodic blood tests at the Radcliffe Infirmary to check on their hemoglobin; none had lasting ill effects. Chemicals in tall bottles called Winchesters were brought up on trolleys via the elevator; sometimes a bottle fell on the floor and broke. The girls had to wipe up quickly, before the rubber composite on the floor dissolved.

The danger of fire in the lab was real but hardly contemplated because there was no alternative way to do the work. So, too, was the threat of fire from the skies. Some nights the girls served as fire watchers, in case an incendiary bomb was dropped, but, as Ruth Parker later noted, "The place was full of inflammable materials. What could we have done with a stirrup pump and a bucket of water? It's ridiculous but at the time it never entered our heads. We were going about at night with no streetlights and our bicycle torches cut by half."

For all this they were paid starting at fifteen shillings a week; after a month it was raised five shillings, to £1. Megan gave half of her salary to her parents and paid one shilling, sixpence for insurance, meaning she had eight shillings, sixpence for herself, or about $1.75. "We had fun," she later recalled. "We went out together—the technicians, George and the girls. We went to the theater and met in each other's homes. Everything was precious at that time. We had to make do and recycle everything we could."

The girls' relationship with Glister was easy and relaxed, and he liked to joke with them. Heatley often dropped in from his adjoining lab; Chain and Abraham, whose lab was on the floor below, made fewer visits, as did Florey, whose office was close by; he later installed a traffic light by the door—green meant it was all right to enter and red, the usual color, meant stay out. While the girls and the technicians called one another by their first names, it was always *Dr.* Heatley or *Dr.* Chain—though the researchers also called the girls by their first names. Florey was always the Professor. They found Florey reserved, Abraham serious and never talkative, and Heatley ideal to work for. Chain, Ruth Parker says, was "excitable. He paced the room with his hands behind his back, propounding his theory with bright eyes and humor. He never entertained us on the piano. You didn't do things like that. Our world was a very narrow sphere and existence in those days." In the evening, Ruth often attended scientific lectures or went to chemistry classes with her brother Donald. To improve technicians' abilities, the Workers' Education Association, in partnership with the university, offered glassblowing classes for making lab equipment and a course in histology, which entailed cutting and examining sections of tissue embedded in paraffin wax.

The girls' sphere was not so narrow that they were unaware of the importance of their work; they knew that success would benefit the troops. Ruth Parker still has "a sense of how special a time that was. Oxford was a special place; the top brains in the world were there. Students wore gowns all the time, so you were aware that they were part of the university. Yet there was a great divide between the town and the university, even though lots of people from the town worked there and trades people got a living." Until recently, the university was the only big employer in town.

The work of everyone from the Penicillin Girls to Florey made a critical contribution to the work on penicillin, and while they shouldered together, the social strata of the lab were unspoken but clear. For the morning coffee break, the doctors and researchers gathered in the library, where refreshments awaited them. The girls and technicians went to the basement storeroom to make their own.

In January 1941, seven months after the first mouse trials, there was enough penicillin to conduct at least a few tests to determine its effectiveness—or harmfulness—in humans and to measure its rates of absorption and excretion. While there was no question that the small amounts required to treat a mouse caused no harm, there was no assurance that a dose large enough to kill a bacterial infection in a human would be equally harmless. Because no one on the Dunn School staff was a clinical physician, Florey went to Dr. L. J. Witts at the Radcliffe Infirmary, with whom he had worked at Cambridge in the late 1920s. Witts agreed to help and assigned Dr. Charles Fletcher, one of his research students, to find suitable patients and administer the shots.

Some scientific pioneers, such as Wilhelm Röntgen with X-rays and Pierre Curie with radium, first test their discovery on themselves. Others feel it is more sensible to test it on a patient who is near death and, after being well informed of the possible consequences, is willing to take an altruistic risk. Either choice is problematic. Florey finally decided on the latter course. One historian has written, "There would have been no shortage of volunteers from the Dunn School staff, but neither Witts nor Florey felt justified in subjecting a healthy young adult to something that might do permanent damage." Gardner, however, was unaware of any such conversations. "I am surprised and a little bit ashamed that none of the penicillin team volunteered to be the guinea pig," he recalled in his memoirs, "but I don't remember even thinking about it at the time."

If penicillin was to be tried on a sick person, the obvious and the most ethical course would have been to inject someone dying of an infection. That was not possible in this instance; if the patient died after receiving the penicillin, the very state of his condition would preclude a determination of whether the death was the result of the drug or the infection. Instead, Florey and Witts settled on finding a patient dying from cancer and who, having been thoroughly warned of the risks, would volunteer to receive an injection.

On January 27, they stood in the Radcliffe Infirmary beside the bed of Mrs. Elva Akers, fifty, of Oxford, who had inoperable cancer and only a month or two to live. Although Mrs. Akers knew that the penicillin would almost certainly neither help nor harm her, she was "rather proud to help in this important test," Gardner recalled. Charles Fletcher injected 100 mg intravenously. Because there had been no report of the work of the Dawson group in New York, it was presumed to be the first time penicillin was injected into a human, and a plaque in the Radcliffe's lobby still commemorates the event.

At first there was no reaction, but, after about two hours, Mrs. Akers had an attack of rigor, a combination of shivering and a rising temperature. The question was whether this was a reaction to the drug or if it was caused by minute traces of contaminants, such as bacterial breakdown matter left in the drug or in what is presumed to be sterile distilled water used to liquefy the drug for injection. Such contaminants are called "pyrogens" because of the fever they cause. Florey, more annoyed than concerned, quickly ran tests and discovered that pyrogens had made their way into the solution; the penicillin was not toxic. A more stringent course of chromatography removed the impurities and Mrs. Akers had no reaction to the next injection.

Within a short time Florey established that because the kidneys quickly extracted penicillin from the blood, the most effective way to maintain a high level of penicillin in the bloodstream was to administer it via an intravenous drip. Assured that penicillin was not toxic to humans, at least in small doses, and confident that the best way to administer it had been established, Florey asked Fletcher to find a patient with a severe bacterial infection unresponsive to any other drug.

Fletcher did not have to look far. Hospitals at the time—as they had been for hundreds of years—were places where people went to die.

"Every hospital then had a 'septic' ward," he later wrote, "filled with patients with chronic discharging abscesses, sinuses, septic joints, and sometimes meningitis. Patients with staphylococcal infections would be ideal because sulphonamides had no effect and were inactivated by pus." The particular horror of septic wards was the ratio of useful care to critical illness: The only treatments for septic ward patients were "bandaging and rest. There was nothing else. About half the people who came to these wards died."

One of the unfortunates in the Radcliffe's septic ward was Albert Alexander, a forty-three-year-old Oxford police constable described by Florey as "very agreeable," who had scratched his face while working in his rose garden on a day off in September 1940. The scratch became infected by streptococci and staphylococci and spread to his eyes and scalp. He was admitted to the Radcliffe in October, but his condition worsened. He was given doses of a sulfa drug for a week that did nothing to alleviate the infection but did give him a rash. Many of the abscesses caused by the infection were drained, but no amount of treatment could save his left eye, which was so infected that it had to be removed on February 3. In the week that followed, his lungs and a shoulder became infected; the bacteria were eating him like a worm in an apple. "He was in great pain," Fletcher recalled, "and desperately and pathetically ill." All the incisions in his scalp, face, arms, and eyes were suppurating, and his lungs were expelling purulent phlegm. Heatley's diary is succinct: "He was oozing pus everywhere."

On February 12, Alexander was given 200 mg of penicillin, the largest individual dose yet given, which was followed by three doses of 100 mg every three hours. Within twenty-four hours there was "dramatic improvement," Heatley wrote, "so they are going to increase the dose." Dramatic indeed: after just eight injections his scalp had ceased discharging pus and that from his right eye and arm were appreciably less. His temperature was normal, and his appetite returned. His urine was collected after every dose, and each morning Fletcher took the accumulated lot the mile to the Dunn School on his bicycle, where the unused penicillin was extracted so that it might be readministered. By February 17, the swelling in his face had nearly disappeared, and his right eye was almost back to normal. He looked well on the way to recovery.

That evening Fletcher carried Alexander's urine by bicycle to the Dunn School, where Chain and Florey awaited news of his condition. Fletcher later recalled "Chain dancing with excitement at the possibility of a real triumph in medicine, and Florey reserved and quiet but nonetheless intensely thrilled by this remarkable clinical story that I had to tell." As Florey discussed what next they should treat, Fletcher observed "the intense joy of the scientist seeing that years of work had resulted in an opportunity to save lives. I remember him saying to me, 'This is the sort of thing that only happens to you once in a life'—and I remember thinking, 'Well, I wish it would happen to me,' and how privileged I was to be taking part in this work."

The stabilizing of Constable Alexander's condition coincided with the exhaustion of the supply of penicillin. Within a short time the equivalent of five doses was reclaimed from his urine but not administered because it was unknown how long treatment should continue after improvement began. Over the next ten days, his condition remained stable, and it looked as though he would fully recover.

On February 22, what meager supply of penicillin had been produced was reserved for Arthur Jones, a fifteen-year-old in the Wingfield-Morris Orthopedic Hospital, Oxford, who had developed septicemia following a hip operation that had required placing a pin in his femur. Over the next five days he was given all the penicillin there was—the five doses recovered from Alexander's urine and what new had been produced. It was just enough to allow him to apparently recover. However, when the pin was removed from his femur three weeks after the penicillin was stopped, the infection and fever flared up again, although he did eventually heal.

Not so Albert Alexander. After ten days of stability, his condition, and especially that of his lungs, deteriorated. A second course of penicillin would probably have had the same dramatically beneficial effect as the first, but there was none to give him. Florey and the others watched helplessly as a flood of septicemia swept through him. On March 15, he died. Florey, distressed by the death, noted the one positive outcome: "The attempt to treat this forlorn case was chiefly valuable in that it showed penicillin can be given over a period of 5 days without toxic effect."

There was a clear lesson in these first two cases, which Florey later described as "typical of those which receive too little treatment. The injections were stopped as soon as there was good clinical improvement instead of being continued until all signs of infection had gone." The challenge was how to produce enough penicillin to treat a patient until all signs of infection had passed.

There was another challenge as well, a double bind that repeats the paradox faced in the early attempts to assay penicillin: a significant quantity was required to meet the standards of proof; in order to convince a pharmaceutical company to manufacture enough penicillin for a large clinical trial, Florey needed to demonstrate convincing clinical success; yet it was impossible to demonstrate clinical success without enough of the drug to give patients all they needed for a full recovery. Somehow, more penicillin had to be made, and Florey had an idea where it could be done.

9

"WILL THESE PLANS
COME TO GRIEF?"

The damage wrought on Britain as it stood alone from the summer of 1940 to the summer of 1941 staggered the country but somehow did not bring it to its knees. Thousands of civilians were killed each month in the attacks on London and all the largest cities—Belfast, Birmingham, Bristol, Cardiff, Glasgow, Liverpool, Manchester. The nation's merchant shipping was steadily decimated; in March 1941 alone, five hundred thousand tons out of a prewar fleet of 20 million tons was sunk. Food was so scarce that each citizen was limited to one egg and a few ounces of meat each week. New clothing was almost nonexistent; heating fuel and gasoline were tightly rationed; alcohol a pipe dream. Perhaps the difference between perseverance and defeat for the British people was as simple yet as powerful as their prime minister's exhortations; Edward R. Murrow said that Churchill "mobilized the English language and sent it into battle."

By April 1941, the demands of war and the bureaucracy of defense had combined to complicate the manufacturing of anything in England. Permits were needed for raw materials, and replacement parts of machinery (when they were available) required the processing of a sheaf of forms that moved slowly through one government office to another. This, coupled with only a small amount of clinical data on penicillin's effectiveness in humans, led to the inescapable conclusion that no English pharmaceutical company would be able to help develop a more effective method of producing it.

Heaven knows Florey did all he could to find a partner. On February 6, Fleming returned to the Dunn School and brought with him scientists from the Royal Postgraduate Medical School and the Lister Institute so that they could see the extraction process. Neither was impressed enough to take on penicillin development. Then in March, Sir Henry Dale, the president of the Royal Society, brought the director of the Wellcome Research Laboratories. Florey was not optimistic about getting Wellcome involved because Wellcome's visit nine months earlier had not yielded positive results. Wellcome scientists not only had been unable to make penicillin in useful amounts, they could scarcely assay what they did produce. This visit did not encourage them to keep trying.

There was one other hope, but it, too, came to nothing, at least for the present. Dale seems to have been the go-between for Florey and Kemball, Bishop, a small chemical company in London's East End that specialized in fermentation. Dale hoped that Kemball, Bishop might quickly produce at least ten thousand gallons of mold filtrate but, between their own war work and the heavy devastation from bombs in their neighborhood, they were unable to help at that point; in September 1942, they would begin to produce large quantities of filtrate that were processed in Oxford.

Florey and Chain were disappointed by these rejections, but they were not completely discouraged because Florey still had one friend to whom they could turn. The Rockefeller Foundation had provided critical support at the start of their penicillin research, and Florey and Chain were hopeful that the foundation would help them again. Because the United States was already helping the British military with its Lend-Lease program, Florey reasoned that it could also help the British scientific community. Besides the foundation's wealth and location in a country not yet at war, Rockefeller offered other strategic benefits. There were many more pharmaceutical companies in the States than in Britain, and, as in Britain, prominent scientists who had high regard for Florey. One mark of that regard in Britain was Florey's election in March as a fellow of the Royal Society, mostly on the basis of his work preceding penicillin, which was as yet unproved.

On April 14, Florey met with Dr. Warren Weaver, head of the Rockefeller Foundation's Natural Sciences Division, who was recuperating in London following a car accident. Florey detailed all the progress the Oxford group had made as a result of the foundation's support and asked for help in getting a U.S. drug company to commit to large-scale production of what he was certain could be an important help in the war. All Florey wanted in return for giving over the information the Oxford group had collected was a kilo of penicillin powder so that he could continue trials of the drug's effectiveness on a minimum of twenty patients and use the results to convince the pharmaceutical companies and the government to undertake its large-scale production. Weaver grasped the potential of penicillin better than had anyone at the British pharmaceutical companies, and he quickly assured Florey that if he could get permission to leave England, the foundation would pay for his passage.

"This project," Weaver reported to New York, "if it were indeed successful, would be more revolutionary than the discovery of sulfonamides . . . and must be recognized as a project of the very highest potential importance. We certainly ought to do all that we can to accelerate its progress."

Florey went to Mellanby to ask for his approval and a few days later received a letter telling him, "The only way that this most important matter may be pursued is for you and Heatley to go the United States of America for three months . . . and get the facilities there under way." In mid-June, the foundation approved $6,000 in expenses for Florey and Heatley, who Florey felt should come along to explain their production techniques.

As with all official travel during wartime in England, the trip was planned with utmost secrecy, and Florey and Heatley were instructed to tell no one about it, even their colleagues at the Dunn School. In many ways, getting the money to travel was the easiest part. There were still exit permits to obtain, other official hurdles to pass over, and most difficult, there were seats on a flight from England to Lisbon and then other seats on the Lisbon–New York Pan American Airways clipper to somehow wangle. Each task required help from high within both the British and U.S. governments. Daniel O'Brien of Rockefeller's Division of Medical Sciences convinced the director of hygiene for the British Air Ministry to give priority to getting Florey and Heatley on a flight from England to Lisbon. Pan American balked when asked to clear seats for Florey and Heatley, and so another foundation executive placed a call to the U.S. surgeon general, who agreed to ask the Department of State for help; three days later, their seats were booked. Beyond the difficulties of finding transportation, there were the perils of the trip itself. Boat travel on the North Sea and the Atlantic was unsafe because of Nazi submarines, and Nazi warplanes were ready to intercept English aircraft flying over Europe, whether or not in neutral airspace.

One night in late April, after he had learned that he was going to the United States, Heatley went with the Floreys and Margaret Jennings to see *Foreign Correspondent*, the Alfred Hitchcock espionage thriller in which a Pan Am Clipper en route from Lisbon to New York crashes into the Atlantic. The struggle of the passengers as the cabin fills with water and their air supply inexorably diminishes is horrific. Afterward Heatley wrote in his diary, "The sinking of the 'Clipper' in the film struck the Professor & me as rather a bad thing to see."

Not long before, Florey received a foreign correspondence that was even more real in its threatened menace. Although the war meant the suspension of publications being mailed between Britain and Germany, until at least 1943, English journals passed into Germany through Sweden or Switzerland, which is how the issue of the *Lancet* with the penicillin report eventually made its way through. A Swiss friend wrote to Florey to say that, as a result of the article, the Germans were interested in penicillin and that they might ask Swiss connections to request a sample of the mold from England. For the last forty years, the German chemical industry had been the model for the world, and Florey held the talents of German scientists in high regard; the sulfonamides were the product of German ingenuity, and Florey had no doubt that if scientists realized the potential value of penicillin, they would turn their considerable talent to developing its therapeutic potential and possibly gain a military advantage.

On April 16, Florey enclosed his friend's letter in one he wrote to Mellanby, saying, "It seems to me very undesirable that the Swiss and hence the Germans should get penicillin, and I think it would be well worth while to issue instructions to the National Type Collection Laboratories not to issue cultures of *P. notatum* to anyone with possible enemy connections. You might also think it worth while sending a note to Fleming and anyone else who might have the mold, although I do not know anyone else myself."

Fleming responded to Florey on April 25, saying, "I am entirely in agreement . . . that we should not pass on cultures of the penicillium to the enemy, and if Ciba, or any other similar firm, approach me I will refuse."

However, Mellanby either missed the implication or was hopelessly naive; either way, he seemed unconcerned that Britain's enemy might gain from the work at Oxford.

"I do not see how the Medical Research Council can ask their National Type Collections to restrict their dispatch of special cultures to different countries and especially to a neutral country like Switzerland," he replied on April 23, but went on to say that Florey should send cultures only "to those whom you feel inclined. It does not seem to me that this is a serious matter, because I expect you are miles ahead of any possible competition." Then he added what could only have been a galling wish, considering Florey's rebuff by every pharmaceutical firm he had approached: "I hope you have been able to arrange for the increased production of penicillin by bringing in industrial interests or otherwise."

There was one bit of interest that Florey was unaware of. On November 29, 1940, an executive of the American parent company of Parke, Davis—the pharmaceutical company whose English branch had produced the vaccines and other products from the Inoculation Department at St. Mary's since the beginning of the century—wrote to a counterpart in their London office. Scientists in the Detroit, Michigan, headquarters had read the *Lancet* article on penicillin and wondered whether Fleming "is in sufficiently close touch with the Oxford group to obtain a sample of this penicillin as well as any information on the strain or strains of mold they have found effective in producing high yields of penicillin. . . . As we are much interested in the direction of effective chemotherapeutic agents, it may be quite possible for us to tie such work in intimately with our present research program."

Fleming replied on February 21, 1941:

I think I told you that the Oxford people make their penicillin from cultures which came from here. In fact, so far as I know, penicillin has not been made from any other cultures. These are now distributed all over the world, and there are many of them in the U.S.A.

I do not know whether I shall be able to get any actual extracted penicillin from the Oxford people, as I know their supply is very limited, but there is no difficulty about the supply of cultures. I suggest that we send him . . . some cultures with complete particulars as regards growth.

I hope to be in Oxford before long and if I can get any of the solid stuff, I will do so.

There is no record that Fleming got any of "the solid stuff" to send to the United States, and he did not pass on the request to Florey. However, Parke, Davis set up a production department at its Hounslow laboratories near London similar to the one at the Dunn School. As Florey's group had not yet published the particulars of their production, the Hounslow operation had to have been based on information Fleming gathered on his trip to the Dunn School. However, it seems that Fleming was not particularly involved with the work by Parke, Davis scientists, who encountered considerable difficulty and soon gave up the research. The only continued commitment to penicillin remained in Oxford.

Even though the production of penicillin was still difficult and any wide medical use still dimly in the distance, it was not too early for Chain to want to patent it. Chain, sick to death of the constant scramble for just enough grant money barely to eke by, was adamant that Florey should seek a patent on their work—not for their own financial gain but rather to bring in money to the Dunn School to more freely finance research. From his father's and his own experiences as a scientist in Germany, Chain knew firsthand how in the competitive world outside Britain patents leveraged economic advantage. His argument with Florey was two-fold: The Dunn School (or the university or the Royal Society, it didn't matter to him) could use the money; and if he and Florey didn't patent penicillin, inevitably someone else would and thus scientists at the Dunn School would be in the ridiculous position of having to pay royalties to use their own invention. In this he was prophetic.

Today it is routine for stock analysts to attend U.S. Food and Drug Administration hearings on new treatments to get the fastest jump on whether to buy or sell shares in a pharmaceutical company based on the approval or denial of its latest products, and a scientist with even the slightest lead on a new drug immediately hires an investment bank to file for an initial public offering in the hope of a patentable remedy. Consider the example of Severe Acute Respiratory Syndrome (SARS). The disease was reported in February 2003. Within eighty days, the Hong Kong scientists (led by a former Dunn School researcher) who first saw the corona virus under a microscope filed for a patent on the germ itself; the Canadian scientists who decoded its DNA filed for a U.S. patent on its whole genome, giving it legal rights to all the virus's genes; and the U.S. Centers for Disease Control and Prevention submitted a patent application on its SARS findings. Each of these applications was sufficiently broad to claim commercial rights in diagnostic tests, drugs, and vaccines.

But this is now and that was then. One of the greatest of the many differences between the German and the British approaches to science in the early twentieth century was the importance of patents. In Germany a patent was a natural and valued part of scientific advance; in Britain it was a repugnant sign of commercialism best summed up by the toast commonly made by physicists working in Cambridge University's Cavendish Laboratory in the early 1900s: "To the electron [discovered there in 1897]: may it never be of any use to anybody." (Which may be one reason why Americans invented the transistor and Germans led the way in science until World War II.) Florey, raised in a scientific culture that revered science for its own sake, believed it was odious for a scientist to claim a gain as his own.

Chain was just as firm in his own conviction: "I could not believe that we would find other substances of equal, perhaps even greater, versatility than penicillin. It was just too much to accept that Fleming had stumbled on the only antibiotic of use to man—the odds of this happening were astronomical. I saw a whole tremendous virgin field and we were the leaders and would remain so if we got enough money. I argued our position again with Florey and we had bitter fights."

Florey remained unconvinced, but he did agree to take up the matter with Mellanby and Dale, the most powerful men in British scientific medicine. Both were appalled by the idea. To them, patenting was unethical. Florey later wrote that their opinion was simply, "The people have paid for this work and they should have the benefits made freely available to them."

Chain's response to this argument was that, "quite apart from economic considerations, in my view it was unethical in respect to the people of Britain, and those of other countries, *not* to protect a discovery of this magnitude for it would then be free for exploitation for any unscrupulous group."

Chain angrily told Florey that he would see Mellanby himself. Mellanby agreed to a private meeting in London but it was a disaster for Chain. In his haughtiest manner, Mellanby rebuked Chain for his crass ambition and, according to Gwyn Macfarlane's summary of a letter from Chain, "told Chain that if he persisted in his 'money grubbing' he would have no scientific future in Britain." Not only would his action "reflect unfavorably" on his own career, Chain wrote in a paper long after he left Oxford, "but on the whole status of my fellow refugees." Mellanby's influence was such that while his implied anti-Semitism was disgraceful, his threat was no bluff; he showed no discrimination in making it clear to refugees and highborn scientists alike that they were subject to his purse strings.

Chain, insulted and humiliated not only by Mellanby's manner but also by an outlook he felt was both stupid and symptomatic of an outdated view of the world, nevertheless had to abide by the decision, even though it rankled him for decades.

"There was a strong streak of anti-Semitism" in England that is summed up in the phrase "Well, he was a credit to his race," according to the late W. Maxwell Cowan. Cowan was a student of Florey's in the 1950s and a pioneer of twentieth-century neurobiology. (He discovered that during the development of the brain, many nerve cells die, and a multitude of other neural pathways are reorganized, thus refining the brain's initial connections.) Cowan felt there were many in English science whose opinion of Chain was, " 'He's one of those bloody aggressive Jews. Probably wants to get rich out of this. That's just not our style.' That was never said but it is fairly clear I think. I saw the anti-Semitism when I was in Oxford."

Florey took it all in stride. His friend John Fulton noted in his diary that "having got his decision from the two top shots in the scientific world he knew he could not be justly accused of quixotic neglect."

During May and June 1941, the third, fourth, fifth, and sixth patients were treated with penicillin, with results that were alternatively promising and heartbreaking. Percy Hawkins, the forty-eight-year-old husband of one of the Dunn Lab's charwomen, had a deep, four-inch-long staphylococcal infection called a carbuncle embedded in his back, and a fever caused by the infection. On May 3, he was given five hourly 200 mg doses of penicillin, then 100 mg every hour following. His urine was collected, and Heatley extracted the unused penicillin that had passed through the kidneys. After four days, there was clear improvement, and his doses were cut in half. This stronger regimen maintained a continuously detectable concentration of penicillin in the blood for the first time. After a week, the carbuncle was almost completely healed, and without the usual scarring. Although this case was not one of life and death, it was the first in which the patient had received an adequate dose of penicillin, and he made a recovery unequaled without the drug.

Florey, both a scientist as well as an administrator who had to find the money to continue, relayed the success to Mellanby and the Medical Research Council:

> I should be very glad if the Council would agree to continue the grant for assistance in preparing Penicillin. We are now employing five girls who are working very well and have been trained to carry out many of the large number of manoeuvers involved in preparing the material. We have just treated a case of a carbuncle with success and without any toxic symptoms appearing. Whatever happens about the future supplies for therapeutic purposes it is highly desirable that this unit, with its trained personnel, should be kept going in order that the chemical side of the problem can be pushed forward with all speed. I should therefore be very glad if the Council will allow me £7 per week for the next six months for the wages of these five girls. At the end of that time

it should be possible to see if any substantial amount of penicillin can be produced elsewhere and the whole position can be reviewed.

Two days later, Mellanby answered:

I think you had better carry on paying the £7 a week to the five girls who are helping in the preparation of penicillin.

I will ask for the approval of the Council at the next meeting, but please don't interrupt the great work.

Midway through Hawkins's treatment, Florey mentioned to Heatley that "an ideal case had just come into the Radcliffe—a boy with suspected staphylococcal septicemia, on which sulphathiazole etc. have had no effect. Could we possibly get enough stuff to treat this case? I said I thought we could." By May 13, however, the boy's condition improved enough that penicillin wasn't warranted.

It was fortunate that Heatley had gathered a supply because that same day four-and-a-half-year-old John Cox was admitted. He was nearly comatose and was so ill that his doctor, Heatley noted, predicted "that he would be in his grave in three days." This dire decline had begun five weeks earlier, when some spots on his left eyelid became infected during what was until then a routine bout of measles. Soon the eye socket was also infected, which led to a cavernous sinus thrombosis, a blood clot in a large vein behind the eye brought on by a staphylococcus infection, which was almost always fatal. Added to this, he had bacterial infections of the lungs and liver, and there also were signs of meningitis. A photo taken upon admission shows John's eyelids so swollen that they look like eggs. As soon as he was settled in a bed, he was given an intravenous penicillin drip.

The youngster touched the hearts of all who worked on his case. By May 16, he was showing improvement, and Heatley allowed an assistant to take the day's penicillin across the university parks to the hospital as "an excuse for him to see the boy."

By May 22, Johnny, as everyone now called him, was talking and playing with toys. Penicillin was stopped, and he continued to get better on his own. Then at one A.M. on May 27, he suddenly vomited and had convulsions. His limbs became spastic and meningitis was confirmed. His temperature rose to 106 degrees, and he slipped into unconsciousness. On May 29, he looked much as he had on admission. Over the next thirty-six hours he was given more penicillin but to no avail. On May 31 he died. His death was a blow to everyone in the lab and the hospital, not just because it looked as though a terminally ill patient would be saved by penicillin but also because he was such a likable child.

Florey, a scientist on the hunt, was determined to find out what had gone on in the boy's head. Had the infection returned? Was there a missed complication? At the time it was difficult to get permission to do an autopsy on a child, but Florey persisted until he had persuaded the parents and the hospital to allow one. Upon examination the pathologist noted "the infection in the cavernous sinus, orbits and in the lungs had been almost entirely overcome, and that the healing processes were well advanced."

What would rightly have been considered a miraculous success instead became the hideous statistic of a cured patient nonetheless dying not from the treated disease but from another cause. John had died not from the cavernous sinus thrombosis, which had nearly been healed by the penicillin, but instead from a ruptured aneurysm in a weakened artery beside his spine.

There were much better results with the fifth and sixth patients, one a boy and the other an infant. The boy had staphylococcal blood poisoning that was unresponsive to sulfa drugs but which was quickly countered by a continuous infusion of penicillin for ten days and then four days of intermittent shots. The baby had a staphylococcal infection of the urinary tract, which was rapidly cleared by small oral doses of penicillin buffered with sodium bicarbonate to minimize destruction by stomach acid. Florey reasoned that an oral dose worked in this case because a baby has very little stomach acid, and because the drug was required not in the blood but in the urine, which gathered a full dose because all penicillin not absorbed by the blood is excreted in urine.

What is remarkable in retrospect is that in the eighteen months of research on and tests with penicillin, the group had used a total of about 4 million units—the amount that now constitutes a daily dose for one person.

While two of the six patients treated to date had died, neither was a failure of the effects of penicillin but rather, in the case of Constable Alexander, the result of their not having enough penicillin, and in the case of Johnny Cox, the result of an unlucky secondary complication. But no serious scientist was going to become excited about a drug in which no matter the reason, a third of the patients receiving it did not live. Still, everyone at Oxford knew they had a medical breakthrough in hand.

Florey also used penicillin topically to treat several surface infections, one being his own case of conjunctivitis. He also gargled crude mold broth on an occasion when he had a streptococcal throat infection. It worked, but, he told his colleagues, "it tasted foul."

"It was clear," Florey wrote, "that substantial doses of penicillin were not toxic to man—in fact one of the most striking features was the improved appetite and feeling of well-being in these gravely ill patients within 2 or 3 days of the beginning of treatment—and there were very good indications that the drug could control the most severe infections. The effect of staphylococcal infections was especially important, as the sulphonamides were of limited use against the staphylococcus." (While a large dose of penicillin is not toxic, repeated use of the drug causes an allergic reaction in some people. Their immune system reacts to it as if it is an invader rather than a savior and creates antibodies to fight it. Symptoms of the allergy can be as mild as small hives or as deadly as anaphylactic shock.)

But Florey's encouragement was the source of his frustration. "The results of this trial were so favourable that further expansion of the work, whatever the difficulties, was imperative," he continued, adding that because of the war there was only the slightest chance of any company being able to manufacture enough penicillin for broad testing. In fact, he realized he was in "something of a vicious circle, for without a more extensive clinical demonstration than had yet been possible it seemed unlikely that any firm would undertake large-scale preparation of the drug, while without a larger scale working it was an almost superhuman task to prepare enough of the drug for the requisite clinical trial." Rockefeller's support would be all the more valuable if that vicious circle were to be broken.

Preparations for the trip to the United States continued throughout the administration of these four treatments. At the end of May, the arrangements were pretty well set, and Florey telephoned Heatley from London to "polish up the bags." Florey estimated it would be another three weeks before all the paperwork was complete. The government instructed Heatley to travel to London to have all the notes and papers the pair wanted to take with them examined and sealed by a censor, who Heatley soon realized quite likely had no idea what he was reading. In these weeks, Heatley collected and freeze-dried as much penicillin as he could, and Florey completed the writing of a second paper on penicillin for *The Lancet*, detailing the effects on patients to whom it had been administered.

The authors of this paper, slightly different than the first, were once again listed in alphabetical order: Abraham, Chain, Fletcher, Florey, Gardner, Heatley, and Jennings—although when it was published on August 16 the editors decided that the running head at the top of the page should read, PROFESSOR FLOREY AND OTHERS: FURTHER OBSER-VATIONS ON PENICILLIN. The summary states: "The work on penicillin briefly reported by Chain and others is here presented in greater detail, and its further development to the stage of human therapy is described." Unlike the short first paper, this one runs twelve pages and describes in detail the growing and assaying of penicillin, the effect of the drug on cells, its absorption and excretion, and the effects on the six patients to whom it was given.

The war, meanwhile, was still going very much the Nazis' way. In June, in the Mediterranean alone, they wiped out the last British troops on Crete and signed the nonaggression pact with Turkey. To the northeast, their army was marching into Russia.

On the morning of June 26, Chain came into the lab, saw Florey with his luggage, and asked where he was going. America, Florey answered, with Heatley and within an hour. Chain was crushed. Even though the trip was intended to boost production, and Heatley, being in charge of growing the mold, had filled three notebooks with meticulous observations on the composition of the media as well as the growth, extraction, and assaying of the penicillin, Chain felt that "the penicillin work was a joint venture between Florey and myself in which we were equal partners," and therefore he ought to be going instead. Chain forever felt that "Heatley plays a very minor part in this story, as far as I am concerned." Florey was matter-of-fact to Chain about the arrangements. The trip was about production, not personal feelings. As Jonas puts it, "Neither man was known for putting sentiment above ambition."

"No other word of explanation came from him," Chain wrote in 1979. "I left the room silently but shattered by the experience of this underhand trick and act of bad faith, the worst so far in my experience with Florey. It spoiled my initially good relations with this man forever."

As Chain's biographer Ronald Clark observed, Florey's character would have made him meticulously follow the need for secrecy, and, although this sudden news was an undeniable shock to Chain, he might have responded with more understanding but for his "unconscious habit of seeing incidents as personal slights when none were intended." Though Florey undoubtedly meant no personal slight, this disappointment came so soon after the argument over whether to patent penicillin that it must have made the blow doubly painful for Chain, and the trip to the United States marked an irreparable downward turn in their relationship. In 1978, Chain wrote to Gwyn Macfarlane, "I always have considered, and still do, that Florey's behaviour to me in the years 1941 until 1948 when I left Oxford for Rome, was unpardonably bad. I could give many examples of this, but I prefer to cover the relevant episodes with silence, as I have done in the past. They were undoubtedly due to human weakness."

After lunch that day, the Floreys picked up Heatley and they set off for Bristol, fifty-five miles away on the southwest coast. "A fine hot sunny day it was," Heatley wrote in the new diary he had packed for the trip, describing "a picnic tea in a beautiful little valley." After a three-and-a-half-hour drive, they checked into the Grand Hotel and, following dinner, strolled through the city, seeing firsthand the "appalling" damage from bombs.

Heatley's last entry in the diary he left behind ends with the details of travel to America: "[We] leave at 7:00 a.m. for the airport, where we embark for Lisbon. On June 30 we are due to leave by Clipper for U.S.A." The final line says everything about what else was unwritten and surely unspoken about the trip and the project as a whole:

"Will these plans come to grief?"

10

THE FRIEND IN DEED

On the morning of June 27, 1941, Florey, Heatley, and five other passengers boarded a Dutch plane at an aerodrome Florey described as "bristling with wire and guards" and embarked for Lisbon. Florey kept his briefcase, filled with mold samples, cotton-wrapped vials of penicillin, notebooks, and the typescript of the upcoming *Lancet* paper, on his lap for the whole journey. As a loose-lips-sink-ships security measure, the windows of the plane were either boarded up or opaque, so there was no seeing out to discern the route. "The sensation was like being in a tube train but less noisy," Florey wrote to Ethel the next day. Half an hour later they landed at an unidentified airfield with a view only of sand dunes and were herded into a hut with no clear windows, kept under guard, then put into another blacked-out plane. After two hours in flight, its windows were uncovered, and they were able to look out for the last five hours to Lisbon, where a Rockefeller representative met them, gave them each $50 in escudos, and took them to their hotel. Determined to take no chances, especially in a city known for espionage, Florey stood by the hotel manager until his briefcase was safely locked away. Each morning he checked to be sure it was still there, and he worried for the whole stay that the high heat and humidity might destroy the penicillin's potency.

For Florey and Heatley, inured to wartime Britain, Lisbon offered unaccustomed luxury; Heatley called it "a freely-lit, non-rationed paradise." Fresh fruit and other delicacies, long disappeared from England or severely rationed, were abundant. "The food I had better not mention," Florey wrote to Ethel. A simple after-dinner walk down crowded and brightly lit streets after what would have been black-out time in Britain seemed strange, especially after spending the previous evening walking in the almost deserted and badly blitzed part of Bristol. Lisbon's dazzlingly white stone buildings with red-tiled roofs were a bright counterpoint to the gray piles at home, and the palm-lined, wide, and what Florey described as "elegantly lit" Avenida da Liberdade with its pavement of patterned black-and-white stones was unlike anything in England. Even the hotel was different: the travelers were given fresh bed linens and towels every day.

As anyone who has seen *Casablanca* remembers, Lisbon was the narrow portal for escape to America and a ticket on the Pan Am Clipper about the most prized piece of paper in Europe. Florey and Heatley arrived at the airline's office on a Saturday, and, to the intense jealousy of several people who had been waiting for weeks to leave, they were given tickets for Monday, evidence of the urgency of their journey.

The flight was delayed by a day, so, on the morning of July 1, they were driven quite a distance up the Tagus River to the base for the Pan Am flying boats and boarded the "Dixie Clipper" through a strong wind from the idling propellers. Baggage and freight that included three hundred two-day-old chicks for a Bermuda farmer were loaded with nearly twenty-four hundred pounds of mail, and, at ten A.M., the plane taxied across the clear water and took off. The Boeing B-314 Clippers were the apex of airborne comfort, as spacious as today's jets are cramped. The passengers—sixty when the seats did not need to be made into beds and thirty-six for transoceanic flights— were spread among six compartments; a common lounge turned into the dining room where meals were served by white-coated stewards and wine was drunk from silver goblets. Each compartment, Heatley noted, was "as big as my room at Oxford, with luxurious seats and a lot of ingenious lamps and ventilating holes, etc. Lovely carpets and upholstery." The flight deck was above them, storage below. Remembering the grisly scene in *Foreign Correspondent*, Heatley was glad to hear the captain say that there were seventy-five collapsible boats on board, each of which could be inflated in a second and a half. Unlike the flight in the film, this one passed in safety and comfort: about seven hours to Faial, in the Azores, for more fuel, then thirteen hours through the night to Bermuda.

"Everyone on board had been very polite and interested in each other," Heatley wrote in his diary, "but it was amusing to note how they became tired as the evening wore on, I suppose partly from lack of oxygen, and just didn't care a damn for anyone else. The stewards made up a number of bunks and we all went to bed." Heatley's curtained berth was beneath that of Catherine Dreyfus, a twenty-one-year-old French movie actress who said her great-uncle, Albert Moissan, was Napoleon's last companion in St. Helena. Poorly paid scientists were not the common passengers on the Clipper. An American woman who boarded in Bermuda had tried to reserve an entire passenger cabin for herself.

Florey and Heatley's wealth was a few vials of powder. Their job over the next several weeks was to persuade tough scientists that purified mold could change medicine.

It was 92 degrees and drippingly humid when the Clipper tied up at the marine terminal at La Guardia Field in New York City mid-afternoon July 2. The seaplane rivaled the great ocean liners for attention by the press; reporters met every arrival. Florey and Heatley told the *New York Times* that they had come on " 'medical business' but would not say whether it was official." They were taken to a hotel near the Rockefeller Foundation in midtown Manhattan, where they stayed only long enough to leave their luggage and make a quick check of the penicillin, which looked as though it had survived the trip, then immediately went to the foundation for a meeting with Warren Weaver. After breakfast the next morning (the air-conditioned restaurant was an appreciated novelty), they were back again to pick up traveler's checks for their stay and to visit with Dr. Alan Gregg, the head of the foundation's Medical Sciences Division. Gregg was a pragmatist, whose feeling was: "We are always more interested in performance with the money we have given than anything else." This was a pivotal meeting, for it was the first chance Florey had to show the top people at Rockefeller what they were getting for their money. He didn't disappoint.

"The Professor spun the penicillin tale in a really expert way," Heatley recorded in his diary, and later added in a letter to Bickel, "I remember him best of all for that performance—and he was so tired after that long journey. He was very lucid in the presentation of his facts," unfurled without notes or interruption in a factual, rather flat tone. Yet rather than make his account dull, the details were so exciting that they turned Florey's controlled delivery into what Heatley called an "extraordinarily moving" account. He explained all the work done at Oxford with the aid of Rockefeller money and detailed the hopes and heartbreaks of the cases of Albert Alexander and John Cox. Heatley watched and listened in awe as Florey showed why he had drawn the devotion of such powerful advocates as Sherrington and Mellanby. "It was unemotional, but still very telling, and in a startling sort of way it revealed the wide grasp of his scientific mind. Even though I knew the subject well, he showed me new facts, and I realized suddenly how great a man he was. . . . I count that hour in Gregg's office as one of the great experiences in my life."

Florey concluded his presentation by thanking Gregg for the foundation's support and, as a validation of all that had been accomplished, handed him a typed copy of the manuscript for the forthcoming *Lancet* article. It was a performance Florey would give to equally beneficial effect on government and industry leaders many times in the months ahead, and they would mean the difference between whether penicillin was treated as a curiosity or as a scientific and medical priority.

The good impression Florey's presentation made on Gregg was evident in the advice Gregg gave to Florey in how he should proceed. Gregg supported Florey unreservedly, and he told him there were three possibilities for getting penicillin made: by direct negotiation with a chemical firm; by a chemical firm under the auspices and with the backing of the government; or by an academic group. The latter possibility was immediately discarded because of insufficient funds and facilities. As for a commercial firm doing it independently, Gregg feared that the firm might eventually impose undesirable conditions if penicillin continued to prove itself. He did, however, feel that George Merck, the head of Merck and Company, whom he knew personally and thought to be very able and honest, would be a useful contact.

As for patenting penicillin, Gregg shared Mellanby's and Dale's opinion that it was wrong on moral grounds. Plus, he added, there was the practical consideration that patentees usually have to spend so much time fighting infringements that they have little time left for research. And at all costs, the "cornering" of penicillin was to be avoided. Florey had been told by Dale and Mellanby that the *Lancet* article was sufficiently public an announcement to prevent patenting in England, but Gregg was not certain that was true in the United States.

The most practical information Gregg offered was a primer on the two opposing factions fighting for control of U.S. government policy on research money and facilities. There were those, led by Dr. Thomas Parran, the surgeon general, who wanted to maintain and improve social services; and there were others, led by Dr. Lewis Weed of the National Research Council (part of the National Academy of Sciences), who wanted them used primarily for tackling defense issues. Gregg alerted his visitors to this political minefield and, Heatley noted, "strongly advised not to get involved exclusively with either one of these parties."

Following the meeting Florey and Heatley took a train to New Haven, to spend the Independence Day weekend with John and Lucia Fulton and not least for Florey to see Paquita and Charles for the first time in a year. Fulton and Charles met them at the station. Charles, well recovered from a recent bout of chicken pox and dressed in a blue suit despite the heat, was "bouncing around cheerfully," Fulton wrote in his diary. "He was quite ecstatic when he finally saw Howard. It was a heartwarming sight." But the secrecy of Florey's trip meant he arrived without forewarning—Florey had called Fulton the previous evening at ten P.M. to say he was in New York—and unfortunately

Paquita had gone up to a girls' camp in New Hampshire only two days before.

After dinner there was a visit from Stanhope Bayne-Jones, a prominent Yale bacteriologist and former dean of the medical school, who was much impressed as Florey unfolded his story as engrossingly as he had in New York. Fulton had not yet been told all the details of penicillin, and, the more he heard, the more enthused he became; that evening he set to work to do all he could to help his friend meet the right people to gain U.S. help.

Fortunately, the Fultons threw an annual Fourth of July cocktail party, and the more than one hundred guests who showed up the next afternoon included the chairman of the National Research Council (NRC) Committee on Infectious Diseases. The fireworks after dinner were matched by the explosive nature of Florey's news. Regardless of the holiday weekend, over the next four days, Fulton telephoned scientists all over the country and was able to arrange for Florey and Heatley to meet with many of the most powerful people in the bureaucracy of the U.S. scientific world.

In doing so, Fulton put his professional credibility on the line. The impressive roster was testament to Fulton's stature and influence as well as his regard for and faith in Florey. Florey, meanwhile, had to be reminded of his predecessor, Georges Dreyer, who was publicly humiliated by the failed promise of his supposed TB cure.

On July 5, Florey and Heatley were driven nearby to meet Dr. Ross Harrison, the chairman of the Executive Committee of the National Research Council, part of the National Academy of Sciences. After listening to Florey, Harrison immediately set up appointments for him to see the council's secretary to avoid any legal or patent issues with penicillin, and to visit Dr. Charles Thom, a mycologist in the Department of Agriculture's Bureau of Plant Industry in Beltsville, Maryland, just outside Washington, D.C. Thom, one of the world's foremost experts on molds and fungi, was the man who ten years earlier had properly identified Fleming's mysterious growth as *Penicillium notatum*. A meeting in Beltsville was set for July 9. An introduction was also set for Florey with Dr. Lewis Weed of the Medical Division of the NRC, to help with any therapeutic testing that might be needed.

Once that whirlwind of meetings was safely bottled, the remainder of the long weekend, launched so propitiously, passed in a pleasant round of introductions, drinks, meals, and reunions. For Heatley and Florey, it was the first time in months that either was able to relax.

Florey had lived in the United States during the 1920s but this was Heatley's first trip outside Europe. After the deprivations of the depression and the hardships of wartime rationing and shortages, America was a land of abundance, and of high prices. Washington, D.C., in July was also a lot hotter than anywhere in England, and Heatley's woolen clothes—mold spores still in them—were a personal sauna. A search for an inexpensive light suit yielded only "an altogether nasty one . . . which fitted me approximately" for about $20. He also searched for a more inexpensive hotel. Although he and Florey shared a double room at the comfortable hotel that had been booked for them, in order to stretch their Rockefeller money Heatley walked around the city until he found another that was half the price but twice as noisy.

Charles Thom was by Heatley's account a man of singular personality. He picked Florey and Heatley up the morning of July 9 and "rushed out of the hotel as if he was keeping the President waiting," then once in Beltsville proceeded to spend the morning "telling us what could have been telescoped into 15 minutes." A few days later, driving Heatley back to his hotel, Thom launched into a soliloquy about "the horrors of drink. The only thing that he had really objected to in England was that in hotels people were never encouraged to drink 'good pure water, decently served.' "

But Thom also knew molds and the latest in production technique as well as anyone in the world, and he proved a good ally. In his first meeting with Thom, Florey was forceful and direct. In early July, the United States had sent ships and troops to Iceland to supplement, and eventually replace, British forces that were stationed there to protect shipping in the North Atlantic, to ensure an uninterrupted flow of arms from the United States to England as part of the Lend-Lease agreement, and to protect Britain from attacks by Germany from the west.

The implications of this were clear. America, Florey said, would not stay out of the war for long, and enough penicillin would make a huge contribution to saving wounded soldiers. But as it was, there would be no way to have enough. Florey detailed the difficulties that the Oxford group encountered in their effort to produce large quantities of penicillin. The best they had managed was two units per milliliter, and as much of 60 percent of that could be lost during extraction. At this rate, two thousand liters of mold filtrate were needed to treat just one case of serious infection. Quantities of this magnitude would require a massive undertaking by a pharmaceutical company.

Thom was certain that a more efficient method could be found. He sent Florey to see Dr. Percy Wells, the head of the Bureau of Agricultural Chemistry and Engineering, who immediately grasped the significance of the work done at Oxford. Within half an hour of meeting Florey, Wells telegraphed Dr. Orville E. May, the director of the Department of Agriculture's Northern Regional Research Laboratory in Peoria, Illinois, a farming community 165 miles southwest of Chicago. A team there was already at work on how best to produce chemicals by fermentation, particularly those that might make synthetic rubber.

THOM HAS INTRODUCED HEATLEY AND FLOREY OF OXFORD, ENGLAND, HERE TO INVESTIGATE PILOT SCALE PRODUCTION OF BACTERIOSTATIC MATERIAL FROM FLEMING'S PENICILLIUM IN CONNECTION WITH MEDICAL DEFENSE PLANS. CAN YOU ARRANGE IMMEDIATELY FOR SHALLOW PAN SETUP TO ESTABLISH LABORATORY RESULTS IN METAL

The reply arrived the next morning.

PAN SETUP AND ORGANISMS AVAILABLE HEATLEY AND FLOREY EXPERIMENTATION DETAILS OF PROPOSED WORK OF COURSE UNKNOWN AND SUGGEST THEY VISIT PEORIA FOR DISCUSSION. LABORATORY IN POSITION TO COOPERATE IMMEDIATELY

On the evening of July 12, Florey and Heatley boarded a train for Chicago. They shared an air-conditioned, private, two-bunk compartment that Heatley found "luxuriously fitted out and full of gadgets," and as night fell they watched swarms of fireflies flicker in the gloaming as the train sped along on its forty-hour journey. Once in Chicago, it was a quick rail trip south on the "Peoria Rocket," then one of America's fastest and most comfortable trains.

They spent the afternoon of July 14 talking with May and Dr. Robert Coghill, the head of the Fermentation Division. The Peoria scientists were not familiar with any of the work that had been done at Oxford, and so they were full of questions. By the end of the afternoon, Coghill promised full cooperation, providing that Heatley stay on in Peoria to get the mold culture started; the Rockefeller Foundation quickly provided a $300 grant to support him there. Coghill also suggested that once the mold was acclimatized to its new surroundings, deep culture fermentation such as that used in brewing beer might produce better results. Instead of growing only on the surface of the medium, mold in deep culture grows, as the name suggests, below the surface as well, thereby multiplying the yield many times over.

In another telegram, May, who was among those who patented a submerged fermentation process on behalf of the Department of Agriculture in 1935, told Coghill:

I KNOW IT WILL OCCUR TO YOU AND THOSE IN THE FERMENTATION DIVISION TO TRY OUT THE PRODUCTION OF THIS BACTERIOSTATIC AGENT IN SUBMERGED CULTURES

The group also agreed that there should be no individual gain from any advance made in Peoria, and they signed a letter of agreement assigning any patents to the secretary of agriculture:

3. It is agreed that in the event any patentable discoveries are made concerning the production of Penicillin in this preliminary cooperative investigation, such patents will be obtained under the usual Department of Agriculture procedure and will be assigned to the Secretary of Agriculture.
4. Any publications arising out of this preliminary investigation will give suitable credit to the parties concerned.

The Peoria lab was a huge building that housed eight different divisions. The scale of the place, enormous under any circumstance, was particularly great compared to the Dunn School lab at Oxford, and in no way as intimate. That night Heatley wrote, "The Professor and I agreed that there were some undesirable features about working in a government laboratory!"

A more troublesome feature was the scientist assigned to work with Heatley. Dr. Andrew J. Moyer was a genius at getting molds to flourish, but he was also an anti-British isolationist who was convinced that Britain was maneuvering America into war. He often muttered darkly to Heatley about "the gutters overrunning with blood," but, Heatley later recalled, "he didn't say whose blood or which gutters." Only Heatley's gracious manner and high competence allowed their partnership to work, and, although Moyer soon turned more kindly toward his English colleague, he would prove to be as unscrupulous as he was talented.

The work began immediately but progressed slowly. The idea was to first grow penicillin as they had at Oxford to try to reproduce the results, and so flasks were seeded with some of the spores brought to America. In England they had bloomed overnight, but for several days in Peoria there was no sign that they had germinated. A possible cause was that the lab's new air-conditioning would not be ready to turn on until mid-September and so the temperature inside was generally above 85 degrees Fahrenheit, far too tropical for spores whose ideal climate for growth was at least twenty degrees cooler. Midwestern summers are relentlessly hot and humid, and the debilitating conditions that had greeted Florey and Heatley in New York awaited them in Peoria as well. When Florey left on July 17, the spores were still dormant.

He wrote to Ethel on July 22:

My dear Girl,
Perhaps you will be interested to know how things are going since I last wrote. We finished up a pretty strenuous few days at the Fultons by being driven to La Guardia flying field to see someone. We took Eg along + he behaved excellently. He had lunch with us + then Heatley

was left in charge + showed him the planes coming in and going out. There were so many of them that he eventually got bored + had an ice cream with Heatley. He didn't seem to get tired + was certainly not crotchety at all. I've heard from various people who have stayed with the Fultons that they both go very well. Eg seemed genuinely to regret that I was going off. Park appears to be enjoying herself in Camp + I gather is in no desperate hurry to see me so I am not going to fuss about it—Lucia proposed to take her away for a weekend but I hardly wish to have the child about if she's not inclined—you know what Park's like. [Paquita does not recall such feelings. "It was always nice to see him, but he was a formal person. The most emotional thing he ever said to me (was twenty-five years later, after Ethel had died): 'I don't know what I would have done without you.' "]

Heatley + I proceeded to Washington sleeping on the train + pressed about. I met innumerable people + eventually it was arranged through the Department of Agriculture that we were to go out to Peoria not far from Chicago to see some mould kings who worked in a new Govt. lab. Hse. So we set off in a stream-lined air conditioned, diesel engined train with all knobs. There was even a folding seat in our compartment. From Chicago we caught the "Peoria Rocket" + rolled up in a relatively small mid-west town. Everyone has been most helpful + decent + Heatley is now going to work out there for a month or two. Everyone thinks I know more than I do + I have to explain I have no official position but it makes little difference. I have literally met dozens of people + drunk gallons of intoxicating liquors—my nose is even redder than usual. I started a few days ago to work north visiting people working on shock + burns—there are vast quantities of them + I shall be a good long time on the job. It is rather tiring with all the traveling + the hotels + cities are very noisy. I get up around 7 o'clock or even earlier as everyone starts at the crack of dawn but go home about 5 o'clock. It is very hot but my clothes are standing up to the frequent laundering pretty well so far. Heatley had to buy a summer suit but sneaked off by himself + from a false sense of economy got an awful thing but I told him it wasn't too bad.

There is a good deal of propaganda in favour of England + the

Allies, far more in the places I've been to than for "America First". I will try to get some photos of the various activities.

While I was at committees Heatley bought your face powder + lipstick but the range didn't seem to be known. He posted off some stuff to you anyway which I hope you get. Will you let me know your shoe size as I have an offer to get some Nylon stockings at wholesale prices. Lucia + another woman who was there wear nothing else. They wear extremely well + don't seem to ladder easily. Send [your response] by airmail.

While Heatley stayed in Peoria to try to brew a higher yield of penicillin, Florey embarked on a round of visits to U.S. drug companies in the hope of persuading one or more of them to brew ten thousand liters of culture fluid and extract the mold, which at the rate it was produced in Oxford would give him enough penicillin to carry out clinical trials on five more patients. In return, he was willing to give an interested company all the information he had about producing the drug. On his visits he also stopped in to see doctors who were doing work on wound shock.

The day after Florey's departure, the spores had still not sprouted, and a "very depressed" Heatley worried that, worse than being slowed by the high temperature, they had not survived the heat of the trip. He was on the verge of sending a telegram to Oxford asking for another culture before deciding to wait a day or two longer. When he returned from lunch that afternoon, there was a trace of germination in one of the culture flasks. "We felt much better," he wrote in his diary after returning from a dinner at Moyer's home, where Moyer showed Heatley and Gita Burkhard, a visiting Swiss scientist, his collection of stones that he cut and polished as a hobby.

After all her male associates were called for army service, Miss Burkhard had been put in charge of the sorbose-producing plant of the pharmaceutical company Hoffmann-LaRoche in Basel. (Sorbose is used in the production of vitamin C.) Freed by circumstance of the opposition a woman scientist's ideas would have usually received in a male-dominated laboratory, she was able to have her production suggestions carried out and soon had sorbose fermentation batches fifteen times the standard production. This success prompted the company to send her to the U.S. branch in New Jersey, to start sorbose production there. She then had come to Peoria to further study fermentation techniques (although she seems to have taught scientists there as much or more than they taught her) and took a natural interest in the problems of producing penicillin. Getting high yields from fermentation was Heatley's interest as well, and the two strangers in a strange land struck up an immediate friendship that at first was centered on science but quickly deepened into a more personal relationship.

Heatley easily settled into life in Peoria, which he described to George Glister in Oxford as a "typical town of the Middle West, and the people are particularly free and easy. It is quite refreshing to be greeted in a shop by 'Well brother, what can I do for you?' or by a restaurant waitress who takes your order and says, 'Arlrightee.' " One shopkeeper "hoped I would return, for he had so much enjoyed listening to the English speech, which he considered most beautiful!" He paid a dollar a week for a bus ticket to take him to and from his hotel to the lab, worked from eight-thirty A.M. until six P.M. or later, as necessary—often well into the night and Sundays—and frequently was invited to lunch and dinner by others on the staff. He had been loaned a portable typewriter before he left New York, on which he typed up his thorough notes with two fingers and sent in long letters to Florey. He also kept the Oxford group up on his latest findings. In his letter to Glister he added:

> The experts here can make our mould grow in all kinds of ways—with pigment and without, and with spores and without, and they can also control the mat weight and pH (to some extent), but so far no great increase in yield of penicillin has been obtained. Sterile chalk added to the medium after sterilization seems to have a beneficial affect, but if you try this, be sure to bake the chalk very well, as it is most difficult to sterilize effectively. . . .
>
> Everyone here is very kind and hospitable, and do what they can to push along the work, but actually I very much miss the help which you and the girls used to give me. The longer I am over here, the better do

I think we did at Oxford to get as much stuff as we did; you and the girls have become quite a legend! . . .

When we could not get the mould to grow at first, Dr Moyer (with whom I am working) who is a great character, said "I kinda figger we shall be doin' some plain and fancy cussin' around here before long."

Perhaps it was the cussing that spurred the spores. By the end of July, the mold brought from Oxford was at last producing; the white fluff of first growth turned blue-green, then the drops of penicillin appeared, though still not as much as hoped. Heatley, engaged in scientific show-and-tell for his first weeks in Peoria, found it "a relief to have the planning of experiments and a lot of the responsibility taken over by Moyer" and over the next weeks devoted much of his time to assaying the potency of the penicillin that was produced. At the same time, Heatley continued experiments to see if other strains of penicillium had an antibiotic effect. While all of them seemed to produce an antibacterial substance, none matched what *P. notatum* was giving.

The first step toward solving any fermentation problem at the Northern Regional Research Laboratory (NRRL) was to see what benefit if any the addition of corn steep liquor to the culture medium brought. Corn steep liquor is a viscous, gluey by-product of the extraction of cornstarch, the ubiquitous thickening ingredient in sauces and baked goods and the medium for starching shirt collars. In processing, the hard outer layer of the kernel is removed by treatment with sodium sulphite. The liquid that results contains both the coat and the starch. The starch is collected by evaporation and the dark brown remainder with a strong taste of toffee is corn steep liquor. One of the chief reasons the lab was established was to find uses for surplus crops of corn and wheat as well as their by-products that would otherwise be thrown away, and Peoria, being in the heart of corn country, was the ideal spot for it. Corn steep liquor is especially messy and difficult to handle, and there was a lot of it to dispose of if it couldn't be used for something else. Fortunately, it is rich in nitrogen, which promotes growth. As early as 1925, scientists had found use for corn steep liquor in fermentation, although there was no laboratory on the scale of the NRRL. And so as a matter of course scientists at Peoria used it, not as Coghill later wrote because "we were smarter or knew more than other fermentation people," but because "we had tried corn steep liquor in every fermentation we ever started."

As corn was not a commercial crop in England, corn steep liquor was not a medium used in fermentation there. The Oxford group used a boiled extract of brewer's yeast as the engine of their fermentation medium. Yeast had grown enough penicillin to show its potent effect but could not produce enough to manufacture it in great quantity. Once Moyer and Heatley had gotten penicillin to grow using the Oxford technique, it was time to tinker with the medium to see if they could increase the yield. Moyer suggested many plans of attack and inquiry, for instance, that lactose instead of glucose be used in the medium because lactose ferments a bit more slowly and would thus help production. Another was to examine the manufacturing process to see whether they were using too many heavy metals, which are deleterious to humans—e.g., beryllium and lead. (Trace amounts of many heavy metals are necessary to support life, but they are toxic at greater levels.)

By August 10, Heatley was spending practically all his time assaying the potency of the penicillin produced. Yet whatever pleasure there was from the work on penicillin was blunted by Gita Burkhard's return to New Jersey; she was the single distraction from his work. He and she, he wrote, "had lived so much in one another's pockets that the prospect of working on at the lab here in Peoria seems awfully empty."

A few days after she left, Moyer showed Heatley how to set up drums for deep culture fermentation. This time, the spores developed overnight, and, within two days, it was evident that penicillin could be formed in submerged growth, although this penicillin had no pigment and the growth was significantly different from what grew in a surface culture.

At least some progress was being made in Peoria. Florey's visits to various drug companies to try to interest them in penicillin production were generally a bust; only Merck and Company, E. R. Squibb and

Sons, Charles Pfizer and Company, and Lederle Laboratories showed serious interest. Florey said that he felt like "a carpet bag salesman trying to promote a crazy idea for some ulterior motive."

One person, however, knew that Florey was both brilliant and without ulterior motive, and no one was in a better position to be of help. Dr. Alfred Newton Richards, with whom Florey had worked in 1926 while on his Rockefeller Traveling grant, was now vice president in charge of medical affairs of the University of Pennsylvania and head of the department of pharmacology in the School of Medicine. Of more importance, he also was chairman of the U.S. Committee on Medical Research and Development (CMR) and therefore one of the few American scientists with the clout to make penicillin a priority. With the probability of war ever more real, the U.S. government created a new bureaucracy to deal with security needs. The CMR was a subdivision of the Office of Scientific Research and Development (OSRD), created in June 1941 "for research on scientific and medical problems relating to national defense" and given broad authorization to enter into contracts and agreements with just about any person or group to fulfill its mission. The OSRD was in turn a division of the National Defense Research Committee, which had been created in late 1940; the alphabet soup of any wartime bureaucracy is a thick broth.

On August 7, Florey and Richards dined at Richards's club in Philadelphia while he listened to Florey's compelling but unvarnished story: penicillin was more effective against some bacteria than any drug in history, but it was hard to manufacture and expensive as well; the small yields to date meant only a few patients could be treated; but with research money and concerted effort, Florey was certain those problems could be overcome. As a pharmacologist, Richards had no trouble understanding what a drug like penicillin could mean in war, and in peace. Although Florey acknowledged that the evidence of penicillin's effectiveness was still skimpy, as far as Richards was concerned, Florey had proved himself fifteen years earlier, and Florey's word was all he needed to hear. The young man whom Richards had called "a rough colonial genius" in 1926 had become even more impressive.

"Florey is a scientist and a scientist like that doesn't tell a lie," Richards declared some years later.

Henry Harris says simply, "Without Richards, Americans would never have taken over production of penicillin." Florey called Richards's action "the pay off . . . from having worked in the States." And so the Rockefeller Traveling grant of 1925 came full circle. Without it, there would not have been the easy reception of Florey and Chain's 1939 grant request to the Rockefeller Foundation, which in turn led to the grant to come to America, and which brought Florey back in contact with Richards, to whom he had first come through the foundation.

Richards wasted no time. He told executives at the four drug companies who had shown interest in penicillin when Florey visited them—those at Merck, Lederle, Squibb, and Pfizer—that now the government was interested in it as well. He made it clear that any research they undertook would be in the national interest and that sharing their results in this instance would not be an antitrust violation, and he invited the executives to join him at an October meeting with Dr. Vannevar Bush, the head of the Office of Scientific Research and Development, to set a course for penicillin research and development.

Richards's enthusiasm and commitment were the catalyst in the development of penicillin and dramatically changed its course, but it would be a while before that was evident. In the weeks following Florey's meeting with Richards, there was no way for him to foresee his good fortune, and so he continued his travels to find someone willing to make him his penicillin for trials on patients in exchange for all the information the Oxford group had gathered.

On August 17, Florey returned to Peoria for two days to check how Heatley and Moyer's work was progressing and to ask Heatley to join him a few days hence in a visit to the Connaught Laboratories in Toronto. When Heatley left on August 23, he was not sure if he would be back in two weeks or would never return to Peoria.

The Connaught Laboratories were nominally part of the University of Toronto, but because they manufactured and sold such products as insulin, liver extract, and various vaccines, it was, to an even greater degree than the Inoculation Department St. Mary's Hospital in London, a wealthy fiefdom unto itself. Among its staff was Dr. Ronald Hare, who had worked with Fleming in Almroth Wright's lab and whose later sleuthing through the weather reports of 1928 solved the riddle of how Fleming's mold could have grown. Hare was astonished by the luxury of his surroundings at Connaught. "The country might be in a depression and some of it bankrupt, but not the Connaught Laboratories." The building was "magnificent," the labs "palatial. One ... was about 30 feet square but, for all that, inhabited by one technician. . . . [The office] was larger than the laboratory in which penicillin was discovered."

It was the very sort of palace that Fleming warned against.

Florey hoped that because of the Connaught's resources and because, as part of the British Empire, Canada was already at war, scientists there would be more willing to help than those in the United States. Canadian soldiers, after all, would be among the first beneficiaries of mass-produced penicillin.

On August 28, Dr. Robert D. Defries, the Connaught's director, asked Hare to join him for a meeting with Florey and Heatley. Neither had yet seen the *Lancet* article published August 16 that detailed the work at Oxford, and so they found Florey's recitation of the facts to be what Hare called an "almost incredible story."

However incredible the story, as soon as the Connaught scientists grasped what would be required for production, "the problem," Hare wrote in 1970, "became formidable. Large rooms would be required merely to act as incubators in which to grow the mould. And the method of purification employed at that time seemed difficult to adapt for large-scale production." Hare and Defries consulted with the chemists on the staff to have their thoughts. "When they asked us how we proposed to produce penicillin, and we told them by growth of the mould in containers of some kind, they laughed at us and predicted that by the time we had spent a great deal of time, money and energy on something so futile, they, the chemists, would have found a way to synthesize it. We must have been unlucky in our choice of chemists because penicillin cannot, even now, be synthesized in any quantity."

The Connaught scientists felt that Florey was asking a lot of them, and that, in any case, large-scale production was under way in Peoria. Florey might gracefully have accepted their decision if that was their sole reason. But Defries further said that penicillin was still to be proved against organisms other than staphylococcus, and claimed that prudence was called for in the face of what proved the vast limitations of the initially promising arsenical and sulfonamide drugs. Yet the first *Lancet* article, which both Hare and Defries had read, clearly showed penicillin's effectiveness against gangrene and other organisms, and the August 16 *Lancet* article, which Florey let them read in the typescript copy he had with him, detailed the use of penicillin against blood poisoning. Also, both Defries and Hare knew that it would take very little more penicillin to test against other organisms and that what was being produced in Peoria ought to help quickly resolve the issue. Still, Defries, for reasons that were never recorded but which a bitterly disappointed Florey rejected as "fallacious," declined to be of any help. Hare felt that Florey never forgave them, and, in the case of Defries, he was probably right.

Defries's zealous caution would prove common. Even as penicillin showed more and more promise in the relatively few patients who were treated, drug companies were leery of committing much money to it because they were afraid of the risks. Gladys L. Hobby, who worked with Henry Dawson at Columbia, wrote in *Penicillin: Meeting the Challenge* that in the case of U.S. pharmaceutical companies, it was fear that penicillin mold would contaminate other products; or that it would be too expensive to produce; or that it would be synthesized so quickly that the cost of manufacturing equipment would not be recouped; or even that when used on a much larger group of patients, penicillin would prove either toxic or less effective than thought.

The Florey road show continued on to Rochester, New York, with a quick visit to Eastman-Kodak and a look at their distillation processes for making vitamin concentrates. Heatley was also interested in a capsule recently developed by scientists there that he thought might allow penicillin to be administered by mouth. Over dinner at the home of one of the scientists, Heatley listened as visiting sisters-in-law "spent their whole time in their small town in N. Carolina in organizing help for Britain. They were just dripping with anti-Nazi venom."

Moyer's isolationism was rapidly becoming passé. America, which had declared itself neutral at the beginning of the war in Europe, was by its continued and escalating assistance of Britain now neutral in name only. From August 12 to 14, President Franklin Roosevelt and Prime Minister Winston Churchill held the Atlantic Conference on the heavy cruiser USS *Augusta* and the British battle cruiser HMS *Prince of Wales* in the mid-Atlantic to discuss strategies of war against Germany and the other Axis nations. While the particulars of those deliberations were secret, the meeting also produced the Atlantic Charter, which in a joint announcement on August 14 the two leaders made known what they termed "certain common principles in the national policies of their respective countries on which they base their hopes for a better future for the world." The eight points of the charter declared principles of freedom, democracy, and collaboration between nations for economic gain; in 1945, those eight points would become the basis of the United Nations Charter.

Florey went for the Labor Day weekend in early September to the Fultons, even though they and his children were not there, while Heatley had a reunion with Gita Burkhard, whom he was happy to see several times over the next ten days. At a party she took him to, one of the guests, "fairly well plastered" he wrote in his diary, told Heatley, "you speak English darn well, you know; not a trace of accent."

Florey prepared for his return to England while he and Heatley wrote a report for Warren Weaver of what their trip had accomplished. Gita Burkhard's return to Switzerland on September 9 was wrenching for both her and Heatley; like many couples who had brief wartime romances, they would never see each other again. He tried to do more work on the report "but felt too bad."

When Heatley and Florey met with Weaver the next day, it was agreed that Heatley should stay on at Peoria until December 16, and the foundation agreed to provide a salary for an assistant. On September 13, Florey arrived in New York with Paquita and Charles, and Heatley joined them for a visit to the Science Museum in Rockefeller Center. The next year, Paquita would ask Heatley to be her godfather.

Fulton noted in his diary: "Howard . . . set off this morning with Paquita and Eg to give them a weekend in New York. . . . The two youngsters are excited beyond belief and Howard a little apprehensive over just how he will keep them in tow in the big city." The next day he added, "Howard . . . returned exhausted just before supper from his weekend in New York with Paquita and Eg. We tried to brace him up during the evening."

Heatley said good-bye to Florey, expecting that they would not meet again until both were in England, and caught the afternoon Twentieth Century Limited for Chicago. On September 14, he was back in Peoria. This trip was not the great adventure of the one in July. Heatley "felt rather depressed. . . . Peoria reminds me of good times in the past. I have the feeling that these three months are not going to be fun."

Warm welcomes the next morning from everyone at the lab, including Moyer, brightened the day a little, but Heatley's gloom persisted for many days. Over the next ten weeks, he and Moyer continued their work and agreed to collaborate on a paper describing their findings, though Heatley noticed that Moyer would cover up his notes whenever Heatley entered the room and was often secretive in his experiments.

The day after his August dinner with Florey, Newton Richards set to work on backing penicillin, and, on October 8, Dr. Vannevar Bush of the Office of Scientific Research and Development presided over the planned meeting with the directors of research of four pharmaceutical companies with an interest in penicillin as well as the Department of Agriculture's chief mycologist, Charles Thom. Richards also was there. The executives, concerned about losing any possible financial edge on penicillin, were generally lukewarm in their response to Bush's suggestions, although Dr. Randolph T. Major, Merck's director of research, expressed the intention of Merck to proceed with production and share information with the other firms insofar as was legally permissible. The others were noncommittal but promised to submit the views of the heads of their companies at a future conference.

Early the next morning, Dr. J. C. Woodruff, the assistant director for Research and Development of Merck, phoned Heatley in Peoria to say that a decision was made at the meeting to move ahead on penicillin as rapidly as possible. He added that there were rumors that the researchers in Peoria were losing interest in penicillin; if that were so, he would be thrilled if Heatley would come to work for him, and he offered to provide him with everything he needed. Heatley declined the offer. He told Woodruff that actually the work in Peoria was going as well as could be expected and in a letter to Florey added that the real reason for his refusal was that "to work in the lab would be to sell out completely to them, and other people seem to be stirring at last."

Penicillin was suddenly a hot topic, one that the drug companies realized could be worth major money, as Heatley learned when he had the opportunity to meet with scientists at the Squibb Institute for Medical Research a few days after the Washington meeting with Vannevar Bush, Richards, and the pharmaceutical executives. Where in the past conversations had been open and spirited, Heatley found that the Squibb scientists had been warned by their superiors not to give any details of their work "for fear it should reach other firms through me. They were extremely polite and nervous and asked only superficial questions, and seemed afraid to follow up the one or two attempts I made to give them useful information. It was quite amusing, really." He later added in a letter to Florey, "The rigid instructions not to give anything away had come from the big shots at the top of the firm, and the research people evidently found this distasteful, particularly Dr. [Geoffrey] Rake [of Squibb], who was distressed and apologetic."

Besides Merck, among the interested companies were Squibb, Charles Frosst, and Pfizer. The Rockefeller Foundation agreed with Heatley that he might be of more help if he left Peoria for a while to assist firms working on penicillin. Heatley visited them in October and helped as he could. He felt that in the day he spent at Merck, where he found the scientists working on the mold "as keen as mustard," he did "more to help production of penicillin . . . than had been accomplished in a month at Peoria" and that scientists at Pfizer "were most anxious to cooperate, if they were able to do so, with anyone concerned, including Merck and other firms. . . . But cooperation was not a straightforward matter, as they would be liable to Anti-Trust laws, which forbid this type of cooperation. (The curious position exists that one Government department is trying to bring pressure on them to make them collaborate, yet this department will not undertake to see that they are not prosecuted by another Government department for doing so.)"

In early November, as Heatley began preparations to return to Oxford in December, he received another offer of work from Major and Woodruff of Merck. Heatley pointed out that he already had told them practically everything he knew about penicillin and that he had no training as a mycologist, as a chemical engineer, or as an organic chemist. Moreover, he didn't know whether Florey was counting on him to "help grow some stuff at Oxford." If he was, then there was no way he could stay. But Florey, sensing that he had a better chance of getting his kilo of penicillin if he had an advocate in place, cabled

WHY NOT GO MERCK SIX MONTHS IF THEY WILL PAY YOU. MORE USEFUL THAN COMING BACK HERE

and both Newton Richards and the Rockefeller Foundation approved of the idea.

"I am very grateful indeed to you for making this fine opportunity possible," Heatley wrote to Florey on November 10. "I only hope you will get a bottleful of the stuff before long."

His staying on made a good deal of sense. Moyer had made the mold do everything except increase the yield of penicillin, and perhaps by working together they could finally succeed. They had, Heatley told Florey in October, "a bookful of data but it is negative." By November progress was being made at last, but Heatley found Moyer was secretive about his findings because, he wrote in another letter, "he has a great mistrust of commercial firms. It will need tact to get the information out as soon as possible. (If it really comes to a showdown, I am certain that Coghill will not back him up.)"

By the end of November, when it was known that Heatley would be moving on to Merck, Moyer was getting an increased if not dramatic yield and was even more secretive, but Heatley was loath "to demand full details now" because doing so "might kill the goose for the sake of a (rather addled) golden egg." Before he left Peoria, Heatley gave Moyer his draft of the paper they had agreed to coauthor, and Moyer said he would send his additions and corrections to Heatley at Merck.

Nor was everything in England going smoothly. Florey had returned home in early October, and he wrote to Heatley that things were not quite as they had left them.

> I arrived back intact on 6th October after a very good passage. They decanted us for a day at Bermuda and I had one day at Lisbon. I arrived on the most depressing day possible: damp low clouds, with the inspiring population of Bristol to admire.
>
> As far as I can see things are much the same here, though the production of penicillin is apparently in a complete state of chaos; I have not yet had sufficient courage to put my head inside the theatre. . . .
>
> *Later.* I have superseded Chain in the brewing department and told the girls to just go on making one brew and then starting again. When this is going there should be at least some supplies of material. As far as I can see at present nothing has been produced during the last three months. . . .
>
> There doesn't seem to be much else of interest as the department seems to be semi-moribund as far as I can see. Whatever you do, go and see the firms who are likely to be making the stuff and try to pick up what their progress is. I hope Rake sends his stuff soon; if you should see him ask him about it.
>
> Hope you are getting results of interest and that Peoria is not too terrible.

Margaret Jennings later recalled why Florey superseded Chain in the brewing department. "There had been a lot of trouble with infection, etc. and [Florey] walked in to find near chaos in the incubation room with Chain wreathed in coils of tubing and dressed in [operating] theatre outfit, quite unable to cope. He was quickly dismissed back to the chemistry room with remarks such as 'not being able to organise a Sunday School picnic,' etc."

Chain's recollection was otherwise. "I cannot recollect such incident. As far as I remember, we did not encounter any particular difficulty. Of course, I have always felt (and said) that a little less improvisation and more professionalism would have profited our work. For instance, counter-current extraction was the standard practice in chemical industry for a process like the one we used for penicillin production, and if we had turned to industry for a commercial centrifugal machine when I asked for it, very soon after we began the extraction process we would have fared much better, and would have saved time." There is little evidence to back his scenario.

Toward the end of November, Florey wrote to Heatley that life at the Dunn School had turned toward normal and that they had made some interesting discoveries. One was that by more than doubling the length of the glass columns in Heatley's extraction machine, a much higher amount of penicillin was recoverable. "We have lengthened the tube through which the drops fall to 14 feet and have fixed up the reservoir bottles on the top landing just before going through the roof. The fall is to the landing of the next floor."

The next week he reported that they were using a different strain of mold than before and that he was sending a sample in case it was useful for Merck. Meanwhile, his difficulty in getting a British pharmaceutical company involved in production was unchanged.

"We had a visit from Glaxo, who were full of enthusiasm. They said we should hear from them in a fortnight; only a month is past! It is a sad difference between these firms and the better American ones, and I do not see what can be done. I am looking forward for the first lot to arrive from America which we can wield about in front of these merchants here, who think we are more or less half-witted."

There was a bit of laboratory gossip, with a passing elbow at Chain: "Since you are not coming back I have moved Abraham [who had been sharing a lab with Chain] up into your room so that all the extractions can be carried out on the same floor. There are also other reasons which I shall leave you to divine."

Four months after going to America to trade all the Oxford group's knowledge of penicillin in return for enough to conduct clinical trials,

Florey was no better off than when he left. Fortunately Dr. Gordon Sanders of the Dunn School staff, whose capabilities for invention and improvisation were almost the equal of Heatley's, came to the rescue. He cobbled together a remarkable production plant in the former animal autopsy room behind the lab.

The morgue elaborately designed by Dreyer was already remarkable: Two giant doors and a more human-scale one opened into a room with eleven-foot ceilings; there was space, Heatley said, "for a post-mortem on an elephant." The walls and woodwork were painted a primrose yellow; two large windows provided plenty of light.

The apparatus Sanders manufactured and assembled, which included a bronze letterbox and a couple of aquarium pumps, was just as incongruous as a dissection room large enough for an elephant in a lab that used animals no larger than a dog. Sanders cut, threaded, and joined hundreds of feet of green, brown, and red three-quarter-inch pipe, along with vast lengths of glass and rubber tubing that centered on eight ten-gallon milk churns. A six-foot bathtub became the holding tank for crude filtrate; trash cans were turned into steam-heated stills; large tanks near the ceiling held amyl acetate; and the mold broth was passed into and through a variety of dairy equipment, including separators and milk coolers. The only pieces of real scientific equipment were two centrifuges. The whole contraption could process 160 liters of mold juice in three hours, then had to be stopped to clear away the gummy residue from the centrifuge.

Elegant in its own way, if not pretty, for the next two years this would be the largest penicillin extraction plant in Britain. But if penicillin was going to make a difference in the war, much bigger plants were needed, and the Americans were building them.

11

THE KILO THAT NEVER CAME

The attack by Japan on U.S. Navy ships anchored in Pearl Harbor on December 7, 1941, and the ensuing declaration of war on the United States by Germany and Italy changed not only the course of the war but also the course of the development of penicillin. With millions of American lives now at stake, penicillin was no longer just a scientific fascination, it was a medical necessity.

Immediately after the attack, Churchill arranged a meeting with Roosevelt and visited him in the White House from December 22, 1941, through January 14, 1942. On December 26, he addressed the Joint Houses of the United States Congress.

The forces ranged against us are enormous. They are bitter. They are ruthless. . . . They have plans and designs which have long been contrived and matured. They will stop at nothing that violence or treachery can suggest. . . .

We have performed the duties and tasks of peace. They have plotted and planned for war. This naturally has placed us, in Britain, and now places you in the United States at a disadvantage which only time, courage and untiring exertion can correct. . . .

Sure I am that this day, now, we are the masters of our fate. That the task which has been set us is not above our strength. That its pangs and toil are not beyond our endurance. . . .

The United States, united as never before, has drawn the sword for freedom and cast away the scabbard. . . . Here we are together, facing a group of mighty foes who seek our ruin. Here we are together, defending all that to free men is dear. Twice in a single generation the catastrophe of the world has fallen upon us. Twice in our life time has the long arm of fate reached out across the oceans to bring the United States into the forefront of battle. . . .

On December 28, Heatley wrote to Florey, "Churchill's speech on Boxing Day was a masterpiece and probably did more for Anglo-American relations than any number of goodwill missions." Heatley had joined Merck on December 16 and wanted to pass along every detail of his talks with various people regarding penicillin. He also had arranged for some corn steep liquor to be sent to Oxford so that the Dunn School group could see what effect it had on producing a richer yield. He told Florey, who was pessimistic about the chances that he would receive his kilo of penicillin anytime soon, that he "tactfully tried to . . . shame Merck into sending you some. . . . I think your fears that none will be sent till the structure has been found and the chemical work completed are without foundation." Heatley now was optimistic about what he might accomplish. "As I told you, I thought I should soon cease to be of any real help on the P problem, as the research staff here are a very smart lot, but actually I think I can show them quite a few tricks and now I have no qualms of conscience in staying on. The large scale production is a terrific problem."

In early January 1942 Florey had a bit of good news. Imperial Chemical Industries (Dyestuffs) (ICI), agreed to help with the manufacture and chemistry of penicillin, but, for the first time, Florey and Heatley found themselves in the position of not being able to openly discuss every aspect of their work. Because of the proprietary concerns of both ICI and Merck, Florey wrote Heatley, "I shall not be free to pass on information on [the chemical] side, and you, of course, will not be able to let me know anything from your side. However, I hope and expect still to get supplies for clinical use from Mercks and Squibbs. Will you please give them my full assurance that any supplies they send will be used exclusively for clinical work and such chemistry as we should be able to do will be done on material locally manufactured. . . . Our tongues are just hanging out for the stuff here and I have made complete arrangements for clinical trials." He added that as far as he could see, the English companies "expect to pick our brains for nothing," and he was willing to deal with any pharmaceutical company in America. "I have no scruples in taking help from wherever I can get it, provided I am not asked to do anything to infringe my academic status and that of the department."

He also asked a favor: "I would be very glad if you could forward me some pipe-cleaners. They are not obtainable here and are very useful for many experimental purposes." And he closed with a slightly envious joke. "People here send their greetings and I hope you have a successful time at Mercks. Your standard of equipment and expenditure will probably be so high when you return that there will be no holding you."

The difference between the labs at Merck, which were equipped with every bit of modern apparatus, and at the Dunn School are evident in a letter from Florey to Heatley on February 6.

> You may be interested in these developments. We are trying to get a milk cooler so that the brew can be cooled immediately after removal from the incubator and the amyl acetate also. We propose to shake out [in] the 10 gallon milk churns, 5 gallons of amyl acetate and 5 gallons of brew. The whole thing is stirred and emulsified, using a gadget used for mixing the cream with the milk which seems very effective. We then proceed to the Ba [barium salt] stage, etc., still using large milk churns. The number of operations is very materially cut in this way, and we anticipate being able to handle about 150 litres a day in about 6 weeks time. . . .

Florey dictated his lengthy letters to Margaret Jennings, who then typed them. They usually were strictly about business at hand, but at the end of this one Margaret added what appears to be the only personal postscript to the dozens of letters written during this period:

> I wonder if you realise that a letter from you is one of the great events of the week in the department? It passes from hand to hand with chuckles (for the incidentals) and excitement (for the major themes). Similarly when an answer such as this is written it involves an hour of

pacing up and down the professorial floor while I sit inscribing in my most rapid longhand (Mrs. Turner [Florey's actual secretary] is almost exclusively absorbed now by the filling in of Government forms)....

We are all almost exclusively absorbed by penicillin now; even shock hardly finds a corner, and seems much less exciting than it formerly did. Did you know that Mrs. Florey is the last recruit to the penicillin team, as she has taken over the clinical side, and is supervising the cases treated, and keeping records, etc.

I . . . have just been home to help celebrate my Father's 80th birthday. The best part of the meagre celebrations permitted by the war was the entirely feudal presentation of an address by the four leading farmers in their best suits and ties; with shuffling of feet and expression of loyalty to the family; followed by a glass of port and slices of cake; and accompanied by the beaming smile of the picture-book clergyman, renowned for his rosy face and his beneficent expression....

We hope we may see you before too long, but not till the useful work you're doing is completed. Perhaps we'll pay a visit to the States to celebrate peace before you come home.

With all my good wishes

Ever yours,

Margaret

Ethel's involvement began in January 1942, when Dunn School workers made the first of what over the next year would be enough penicillin to treat fifteen seriously ill patients and another 172 infections of the eye and other localized areas such as the mastoid cavity of the inner ear. Howard later complained that some of the patients given to Ethel were from doctors who had tried and failed with every course of medicine, leaving Ethel "a corpse retriever." Which actually wasn't such a bad thing, as it made penicillin's success even more impressive. The overriding lesson Ethel learned from all these cases, she wrote in *The Lancet* in 1943, was "it is useless to apply penicillin unless the whole infected area can be reached." A small amount of the penicillin was shared with Flight Lieutenant D. C. Bodenham of the Royal Air Force. His effective treatment of severely burned airmen revealed another aspect of penicillin's power against infection.

While Ethel conducted clinical trials, Florey wrote to John Fulton that now he was "having to do a good deal of the penicillin extracting myself as I found that the girls and the technician who had done a lot of the work with amyl acetate were somewhat anemic and had indications of leucopoenia [an abnormal decrease in the number of white blood cells], so I have had to switch people about and now have to rot my own bone marrow."

For all this time and for months to come, Florey was on the lookout for his kilo of penicillin in the same way that a castaway scans the horizon for sight of a rescue ship. One morning in April 1942, he arrived at his office and thought that at last his ship had come in. The next day he wrote Heatley,

Firstly, thank you for the 5g. [seventeen one-hundredths of an ounce] of penicillin. Will you convey to the right quarters at Mercks my appropriate thanks? For your ear alone I was rather amused at the parcel which arrived in a damn great box which looked as though it might have a kilo in it. This illusion was destroyed when I lifted the box. Inside the box was a smaller box and inside this box there was an enormous amount of packing material encasing the precious material. It was the sort of package in which you might expect to have the Kohinoor diamond.

Florey's kilo was never to be. This literal pinch was the only penicillin sent from the United States for the Dunn School tests. Whatever deal was struck in the summer or fall of 1941 was nullified by America's entry into the war, though no one ever told Florey point-blank that there would be nothing for him. Instead, as the year passed, there were promises for the future and excuses for the present, the silliest being that to keep its potency, penicillin had to be transported in dry ice, but as that would evaporate before the package reached Oxford, there was no point in sending any.

"This of course we regard as grotesque," Florey wrote to J. H. Burn, the Oxford Professor of Pharmacology, "as we keep our [dried] material at room temperature on a bench in the desiccator [used for drying out the powder from the broth] or in a bottle in my desk. I have sent some out to the Middle East [to Colonel Robert Pulvertaft in Cairo, to test on battle casualties] that has arrived apparently quite active. . . . Clearly if it were so unstable as that it would be of very little use."

The real reason, of course, was that the Americans wanted to use every bit of penicillin they produced for their own research and treatment, and Florey added that he knew it firsthand. "I saw Perrin Long [the chairman of the Committee on Chemotherapy] not so long ago and his reason was that the American Government had taken over the stuff."

To promote the development of penicillin in America, the U.S. government encouraged drug companies to collaborate in their work without fear of potential antitrust violations. In February 1942, Merck and E. R. Squibb and Sons signed an agreement to share research and production information. They also agreed to joint ownership of their inventions and to include in this agreement "other firms who have made definite contributions to the solution of the problem." In September, Charles Pfizer and Company, which had worried that penicillin spores would infect the citric acid that was a mainstay of their business, joined the group.

During Heatley's first months at Merck, balky mold slowed production. It was March before the company had enough penicillin to treat even one patient, but that one patient needed it very badly.

On March 12, as Anne Miller lay dying in the Yale hospital and Fulton lay in a nearby room with a serious viral infection, their doctor, John Bumstead, asked Fulton if he would help get some penicillin for her. Fulton sent a telegram to Heatley, describing her illness and asking whether any penicillin could be sent to New Haven. Heatley passed on the request to Merck's medical director, who said that their supply was under the control of Newton Richards, the chairman of the Committee on Medical Research. Fulton telephoned around until he found Richards in Washington, D.C. Richards said that the decision was actually up to Dr. Perrin Long, the chair of the Committee on Chemotherapy. After Fulton talked with him, Long authorized the release of 5.5g for the first clinical trial in America.

The penicillin arrived at the hospital on Saturday, March 14, but as it came with no instructions on how to administer it or what dose to give, Bumstead had no idea what to do. Every doctor at Merck he tried to reach by phone was away, and so eventually he spoke with Heatley, who gave him directions.

Mrs. Miller was listless but aware enough to be worried that the intern who was about to give her the shot "could not get into my poor over-worked veins" with the cruder syringes and broader, blunter needles of the day. She need not have worried. He turned out to be a genius of a needle man.

Mrs. Miller's temperature was 105.5 degrees F (40.8 degrees C) when she received her first injection. By the next morning, it was normal for the first time in a month, and her blood cultures showed that in twenty-four hours the number of bacterial colonies had dropped from 100 to 150 per cubic centimeter to one colony per cubic centimeter. Also, her appetite returned, and she was able to eat a hearty meal for the first time in thirty days.

Bumstead phoned Heatley every day to report Mrs. Miller's progress. In light of her quick turnabout, Bumstead wanted to reduce the dose, but Heatley, remembering the case of Constable Alexander, urged him not to.

These conversations were exciting in their good news and amusing in the little dance that accompanied them. Each day Bumstead asked Heatley, "What would you recommend? Should we carry on with the penicillin?" And every time, Heatley answered, "Look, I'm not medically qualified. It would be quite unethical for me to suggest anything." So Bumstead would ask, "Well, what do you think Dr. Florey would say?" And Heatley would answer brightly, "Oh, I think he would say carry on. You know, you can't stop it now."

On March 19, the penicillin was nearly exhausted, and an urgent call went out for more; Heatley scrambled to get it out that day. On March 22, eight days after treatment started, he visited Bumstead and Mrs. Miller. That night he wrote in his diary that despite all his work with penicillin, he found "the temperature charts, records, and patient's own statements . . . amazing." Almost equally amazing was "a rumor that Mrs. Miller's symptoms had been cabled to England and that someone (presumably the Professor) had made up some shots which had been flown here by bomber!"

Heatley returned to New Jersey with a glass jar full of Mrs. Miller's urine so he could extract the penicillin that had passed into it, and he continued to help make more of the drug. On March 25, another emergency call came for more. Merck's production of enough penicillin to see her through her complete recovery in April ensured the reclamation of her life. (Merck also provided the penicillin for many people badly burned in the horrific fire at the Coconut Grove nightclub in Boston in November 1942.)

While pharmaceutical companies like Merck concentrated on penicillin production, scientists in Peoria continued to search for the fastest way to grow the greatest quantity. Not content to think that they were using the ideal strain of mold, Dr. Kenneth B. Raper, the mycologist at the Northern Regional Research Laboratory, and his staff grew and tested thousands of the many different strains in the *Penicillium notatum chrysogenum* group gathered from soil samples that the U.S. Army Transport Command flew in from all over the world. For much of the time they worked ten hours a day, seven days a week. All molds that showed useful activity were sent to the drug companies working on penicillin.

Of all the samples collected across the globe, none was as good as the one found only a mile or two from the lab. Every day Raper sent an assistant, Mary Hunt, to search the local markets and bring back decaying fruit and anything else with fungal growth, which earned her the inevitable nickname "Moldy Mary." On one of these expeditions she found a cantaloupe with a mold so powerful that in time it became the primogenitor of most of the penicillin produced in the world.

At the end of June 1942, Heatley prepared for his return to England and was able to gather about half a gram of penicillin for Florey. He had yet to receive Moyer's corrections for their joint paper on the work in Peoria and never would; shortly after Heatley returned to England, Moyer submitted the paper under his name alone. Heatley later described this "as something of a betrayal, but the important thing was to get the Americans interested."

During his last few days in America, Heatley took a little time for personal pleasure. He saw his first Broadway play, and made a visit to Coney Island, the famous amusement park in Brooklyn. Ever the scientist, even at play, he decided to ride on a roller coaster called

"The Tornado" to compare it with one in England. He found "it was a bit more vigorous, and though I felt alright when I got off, I began to feel sick and to have a headache minutes later."

The executives and Heatley's colleagues at Merck gave him a fond farewell, and, at the end of the month, he embarked on a less luxurious return to England, as one of five passengers on a freighter. After leaving New York Harbor, the boat anchored off Long Island until it could join a convoy of more than forty ships for the dangerous crossing of the Atlantic. On July 2, the first full day at sea, Heatley took stock of the past twelve months in his diary.

"Exactly a year ago today the Professor and I arrived in America. It has been a wonderful year and I suppose I ought to feel pleased with the work I have done. Actually I have not got such a burningly urgent impulse to get on with penicillin as when I came, but this is probably due to the fact that the problem calls for specialists now in every field." This was especially true in unraveling penicillin's chemistry.

The next day he noted, "There were about eight ships less in the convoy than last night, but we did not know whether they had straggled behind or whether some harm had befallen them. We were told a good many depth charges were let off astern, but none of us passengers heard them."

He arrived safely in Scotland on July 17. The ship was suddenly ordered to make a quick turnaround, and so everyone was hurried off. Heatley rushed belowdecks to recover the penicillin he had stored in a large refrigerator, "which I got after clambering over slippery meat, etc." He took a slow and crowded overnight train to Oxford, which "was dull and very cold and everything looked drab," but dinner with Ethel and Howard made for a warm return.

In the year Heatley was away, rationing grew more stringent in Britain. At the time Mrs. Miller was being treated in New Haven, Florey was vexed by the rigmarole involved to obtain even the simplest item for the lab. The lengths to which he had to go may seem quaint in retrospect, but they were maddeningly frustrating at the time. For instance, in March 1942, Florey arranged for a specialist in molds to search for other naturally occurring antibiotics, but the man needed rationed gasoline for his car. A lengthy explanation and appeal to Dr. A. Landsborough Thomson of the MRC ended:

> He is going to see the petrol controller next week and . . . his chance of being able to get this necessary allowance would be greatly enhanced if he could have some sort of chit from you to say that this work is supported by the Medical Research Council. . . .
> Sorry to trouble you in this way but there seems nothing else to do.

Florey received the chits for the gas, but his troubles were not over. In June, in the midst of "investigating the antibacterial substances contained in plants . . . for their possible therapeutic uses," Florey wrote again to Thomson: "I am afraid I have to trouble you once more for these interminable chits" so that "Mrs. Osborn, a botanist who is doing the investigation and who is the wife of the Sherardian Professor of Botany at Oxford," can have five gallons of gas "to go out into the country in the neighborhood to obtain specimens."

Then in August, after thanking an official of the MRC "for the chit for the iron," Florey wrote, "We are now in trouble as we are not allowed sufficient amyl acetate to carry on our extraction. We are allowed 10 gallons per month and we are using it at a rate of 20 gallons." Was it possible for "some form of chit to try to get 20 gallons per month out of the Control people?"

The necessity to beg for even the smallest items continued well into 1943; on March 27, Florey asked Thomson "if you could give me one of the necessary letters to obtain a bit of timber? . . . The amount required is quite small, it is only £2 worth, but we are unable to get on with setting up the better penicillin extraction apparatus without it."

Despite these bureaucratic hurdles, the Oxford team continued to make progress. On August 2, Florey wrote his old friend and mentor Charles Sherrington, "There is, for me, no doubt that we have a most potent weapon against all common sepsis. My wife is doing the clinical work and is getting astonishing results—almost miraculous, some of them." Yet he was frustrated by the lack of government support. "I am afraid the synthesis of the substance is rather distant," he continued, "but if, say, the price of 2 bombers and some energy was sunk into the project, we could really get enough to do a considerable amount."

The Americans had already made that commitment. By the end of 1943, the production of penicillin was the second highest priority at the War Department. Only the development of the atom bomb was considered more important.

How the name of one person associated with a great discovery rises above another's can have less to do with contribution than it does with the way the story is first told. Certainly that was the case with Fleming and Florey and the others at Oxford. In the matter of penicillin, case No. 12 of the 187 patients treated in England during 1942 and 1943 set the course for decades of misplaced credit for its development.

On August 5, 1942, Fleming telephoned Florey to seek help for Harry Lambert, a fifty-two-year-old friend. For nearly two months Lambert had languished with an illness that resembled meningitis but was not accompanied by high fever; it was unresponsive to every treatment given, including sulfa drugs, and in all this time Lambert's doctors were unable to make a diagnosis. Finally, Fleming ran some tests on a sample of Lambert's cerebrospinal fluid and found streptococcus. He cultured some of the bacteria with a sulfa drug and cultured the rest with crude penicillin mold juice he still produced in his lab. The sulfa drug did nothing; the penicillin killed the germ. Fleming had solved the riddle just in time: that night Lambert had to be put on oxygen and given a heart stimulant.

Fleming asked Florey if he could spare some of his supply of the drug. Florey agreed on the condition that Fleming allow the case to be included in the clinical trials of the Oxford penicillin. He then took all he had on hand to London and showed Fleming how to administer it. Beginning on August 6, injections were given every two hours, and the following day Lambert was improved but far from healed. Despite another forty-eight injections over the next five days of additional material sent by Florey, he got no better. On August 13, Fleming reasoned that if he injected penicillin directly into the sheath of the spinal cord, it would be transported to the site of the infection, and he called Florey for his opinion. Florey told Fleming he would experiment on an animal and let him know the result.

Fleming, however, his skill with a needle undiminished and Lambert perilously ill, decided to take the risk rather than wait. A few hours later, Florey called to say that Fleming should not give the injection—the rabbit he had tried it on died almost immediately. Lambert, however, had no ill effects. Over the next week Fleming gave him four more shots in the spinal sheath as well as others intramuscularly. Fleming was either extraordinarily lucky or extraordinarily precise; today such injections are considered far too risky because it has been shown that penicillin is toxic to the spinal cord and the brain, which probably is why Florey's rabbit died.

Ignorance favored Lambert, and Fleming. His improvement, Fleming wrote to Florey on the August 16, was stunning.

> I am rather a pessimist but it really seems to me that Lambert (the penicillin patient) is going to recover. No temperature—brighter in every way—pulse better. . . . When you saw him he was a dying man. When you see him on Tuesday you will (unless things change) see an enormous difference.

On August 28, Lambert was out of bed and symptom-free. "The patient is very well and appears bacteriologically cured," Fleming wrote to Florey:

> Temperature normal; blood count normal. The only thing he suffers from now is a certain amount of headache. . . .
> I am sending you back 4 c.c. of the penicillin. This is all I have.
> We are all here very grateful to you for your kindness in letting us have penicillin which has in this case undoubtedly saved the man's life.

These letters mark the last days of what for years had been a pleasant and respectful relationship; the two men stand next to each other in a group photo taken outside the Dunn School of the 1932 meeting of the Pathology Society of Great Britain and Ireland. Those days were past. Before long, Florey would lose all regard for Fleming.

12

THE LAUREL WREATH
OF CREDIT

A three-hundred-word editorial in the August 27, 1942, *London Times* seconded the plea in a recent *Lancet* article that the government promote the industrial production of penicillin. Entitled "Penicillium," the article described the "strong antibacterial powers" of the mold discovered "some thirteen years ago," and it cited current work in Oxford that showed the drug was not toxic, was "many hundred times as active as the sulphonamides," and was able to overcome bacteria the sulfonamides did not affect. No scientists were named. "The prospect is certainly an alluring one," the article said and, quoting *The Lancet*, "in view of its potentialities, methods for producing penicillin on a larger scale should be developed as quickly as possible." As *The Lancet* had a readership limited almost exclusively to scientists, the *Times* was the first to widely publicize news of penicillin. The next day the *News Chronicle* had an article on it, followed by one in the *Sunday Express* on August 30.

It was not chance that Lambert's recovery coincided with this sudden attention to penicillin. It had been two years since the Oxford group's first *Lancet* article and one since the follow-up that detailed its effects on the initial six patients. Throughout 1942, Ethel's use of penicillin had cured people, some almost as sick as Lambert, but there had been no attention in the press. Which suited Florey just fine. There was so little of the drug and still so much to learn about its clinical value that, to him, wide public knowledge would lead to wide public demand that could not be met. Fleming, however, talked about Lambert with his colleagues at St. Mary's, and someone there who did not share Florey's wariness of publicity alerted the *Times,* which on August 31 printed this letter:

Sir,—In the leading article on penicillin in your issue yesterday you refrained from putting the laurel wreath for this discovery round anybody's brow. I would, with your permission, supplement your article by pointing out that, on the principle of *palman qui meruit ferat* [honor to one who earns it], it should be decreed to Professor Alexander Fleming of this research laboratory. For he is the discoverer of penicillin and was the author also of the original suggestion that this substance might prove to have important applications in medicine.

I am, Sir, yours faithfully,
Almroth E. Wright
Inoculation Department, St. Mary's Hospital,
Paddington, W.2, Aug. 28

It is ironic that Wright, who fought with Fleming over his insistence to include the phrase "this substance might prove to have important applications in medicine" in his 1929 paper, now lauded his foresight, but it also is easy to understand why he did. St. Mary's relied on donors for its support, and something as remarkable as penicillin would mean bigger donations if the hospital claimed its place in the drug's development.

Reporters flocked to St. Mary's to interview Fleming, and several stories appeared over the next couple of days. The one in the September 1 *Daily Mail* began:

Experiments in a laboratory at St. Mary's Hospital, Paddington, are being made with a substance called penicillin, which may become the most valuable drug of the war and one of the most important medical discoveries of all time. . . .

Professor Fleming said yesterday: "The production of the drug is very complicated and the difficulties are great, but they are being overcome. I think it will soon be possible to produce it on a commercial scale."

There was a critical error in the story: The experiments were not being done at St. Mary's by Fleming; they were being done in Oxford by Florey and his team.

The headlines in the papers were sensational: "Miracle from Mouldy Cheese"; "Fungus May Fight the Germs"; "New Drug Will Check Infection from Wounds"; "Professor's Great Cure Discovery"; and in the *Glasgow Herald*, "Scottish Professor's Discovery." None of the stories mentioned Florey, but one did mention "research chemists in Oxford."

Then on September 1 came another letter in the *Times:*

Sir,—Now that Sir Almroth Wright has so rightly drawn attention to the fact that penicillin was discovered by Professor Alexander Fleming and has crowned him with a laurel wreath, a bouquet at least, and a handsome one, should be presented to Professor H. W. Florey, of the School of Pathology of this university. Toxic substances are produced by the mould alongside penicillin and Florey was the first to separate "therapeutic penicillin" and to demonstrate its value clinically. He and his team of collaborators, assisted by the Medical Research Council, have shown that penicillin is a practical proposition.

I am, Sir, your obedient servant,
R[obert] Robinson
Dyson Perrins Laboratory, Oxford University, August 31

This time newspapermen rushed to Oxford, but there was not the open welcome they received at St. Mary's. Florey, horrified by the prospect that publicity would raise the hopes of thousands of patients who might benefit from penicillin when, in fact, it likely would be years before there was enough to give any of them, refused to meet the reporters and had his secretary send them away with the hint that if they returned the following Thursday, he "may give them ten minutes."

In an ideal world this was the right decision. By all the standards of science at the time it was the right decision. By the standards of Fleet Street, however, it is hard to imagine a worse one. Given the choice of writing about an unprepossessing Scotsman who willingly received the press or about an unavailable and apparently ill-tempered Australian and his Continental cohort, the gentlemen of the press did not hesitate to decide.

At first, Fleming appeared to do his best to distance himself from the commotion. On September 2, he wrote Florey:

> I was very glad to see Robinson's letter in the *Times* this morning. Although my work started you off on the penicillin hunt it is you who have made it a practical proposition and it is good that you should get the credit.
>
> You are lucky in Oxford to be out of range of the reporters. They are a persistent lot and I have not been able to dodge them completely. I do not know whether you saw the *Daily Mail* yesterday. They started the day before by ringing up Sir Almroth and asking him to write an article for them. They were told we did not want any further publicity. An hour after a reporter arrived to see me and was told I was out. Late in the afternoon this same reporter got me on the telephone and asked me whether anybody in this country was going to manufacture peni-cillin. I said "yes." Then she asked when it was likely to be available and I said "god knows." The result was that in the paper it was reported that I said it would be produced in quantity in a short time. I think we successfully choked off all the others including the B.B.C.
>
> The man Lambert is very well and will be going home very soon. I am writing up a full report from which you will be able to extract what you want for your paper. I am glad you are going to publish your results soon as it may further stimulate the manufacturers.
>
> If you are in London I should like very much to see you as a certain thing has happened which may have an important bearing on the large scale production. I do not want to do anything without consulting you.

Meanwhile, the barrage of stories about Fleming continued. On Saturday, September 5, the *News Chronicle* offered a profile of Flem-ing as their "Man of the Week."

> A man almost unknown by the general public; a tall, slim, grey-haired, blue-eyed man, working in the reek of drugs; a man whose personal

modesty is so great that he refuses to sit for a picture or even to publish his age in works of reference: that is Alexander Fleming, on whose brow Sir Almroth Wright has, in his own words, "placed the laurel" for the discovery of Penicillin, the new wonder-drug.

Up at Oxford, in the Sir William Dunn School of Pathology, a little band of scientists, numbering several nationalities, are working day in and day out, to produce this substance in quantity.

It had taken the popular press less than a week to effectively decide who would receive the credit for penicillin. Fleming was tall [only in his newfound stature; he was still just over five-foot-five], slim, gray-haired, blue-eyed, and modest. Florey, Chain, and Heatley were anonymous members of a little band of foreigners.

On September 7, Fleming again wrote to Florey:

You cannot deplore the personal element which has crept into penicillin more than I do and for the moment I am the sufferer. I was out . . . all last Friday and when I got back in the late afternoon Wright told me that he had been rung up by some weekly review that he had never heard of. On Saturday morning when I arrived in the lab I found the *News Chronicle* planted on my bench. I hated it and have been suffering since. The photograph looks as if I was really suffering—where it came from I have no idea but it is not one I myself would have chosen.

The *Illustrated London News* rang up last week and said they were publishing an article on penicillin. I was told this had been carefully prepared from our published articles and there was none of the daily press ballyhoo. They wanted a photograph of myself which was refused but I gave them some mould cultures to illustrate the article as this seemed on a higher plane than the daily papers. It would be better if it were impersonal but after the letters in the *Times* it is likely that we will be mentioned. [In the article, Fleming mentions "the Oxford group."]

I do hope that the people who matter (the others do not count) do not think that we are in opposition. I will certainly do what I can to dispel the idea that it exists. As you say our contributions are perfectly clear cut and complementary and no one can accuse me of ever having said that my work was not acknowledged.

The only thing that pleases me is that the advances in this direction have been independent of professional mycologists.

When you were talking to me about large scale production of penicillin you said that this was a thing which one of the ministries ought to take up as a war measure. It is in this connecxion [*sic*] that I want to see you.

As penicillin's success became more evident, the greater the acclaim heaped on Fleming. Florey, Chain, Heatley, and others at Oxford remained invisible and unannounced to the public, and for years they watched with dismay as credit accrued at St. Mary's but little came to the Dunn School. Yet Florey could do nothing to counteract this imbalance; besides his distaste for publicity, there was his concern that stories about penicillin would lead to a demand that could not be filled. Plus there was the general prohibition in Britain against doctors' using their discoveries for personal advancement.

Fleming made a separate peace with these issues. From the day that Wright's letter appeared in the *Times*, he was almost constantly available for interviews. In fairness, it must be said that he did not make claims beyond the work he actually did, and many times he mentioned the work done by the Oxford group and others. In fairness it also must be said that having done that, Fleming did not try to correct the record when reporters gave him more credit than he deserved. Fleming kept a scrapbook he wryly labeled "Fleming Myth," which he filled with the scores of articles that appeared. He "positively enjoyed" the greatest inaccuracies, "an attitude" his biographer Gwyn Macfarlane suggests was "perhaps characteristic of his peculiar sense of humor." According to Macfarlane, Fleming viewed even the most preposterous stories with "amused detachment."

The misinformation and exaggerations were repeated for decades and reached either an apex or a nadir in *Alexander Fleming and Penicillin* (1974) by W. Howard Hughes. Hughes, a bacteriologist at St. Mary's from 1936 until 1970, and who therefore ought to have known better, claimed that St. Mary's grew larger amounts of mold than Oxford (in fact they grew none at all), and that "our technicians had been making it every week since its discovery." The broth, he added, was sent in "large churns" to Oxford, where it was turned into penicillin. According to Hughes (who appears to have written in the fog of myth rather than act with malice), it was at St. Mary's that the drug saved the first patient—an unnamed police sergeant who seems based on Albert Alexander, the Oxford policeman treated by Florey in 1942, who, in actuality, died from an insufficient supply of penicillin.

Nor did anyone at St. Mary's step forward to correct the ever-growing record of misattributions repeated so often that they became gospel. It is easy to see why. Chain later said with some amusement, "The British hospitals were struggling for their pennies . . . then here, suddenly, was a pot of gold for St. Mary's. It was an opportunity to be grasped—and if I had been the manager of the hospital, I might have done the same."

Two of St. Mary's most dedicated backers, Almroth Wright and Fleming's old acting partner Lord Moran—who now was Winston Churchill's personal physician and not incidentally the former dean of St. Mary's Medical School—were well connected to the press and, in Wright's case especially, not shy when it came to self-promotion. Fleming and St. Mary's certainly deserved some of the credit for penicillin. If Florey wasn't going to stake a claim for the remainder, they were happy to fill the void.

The British medical historian David Wilson has pointed out, "Florey, well known in academic circles as a tough bargainer when it came to fighting for research funds, allowed the credit . . . to slip away through his disdainful treatment of the media. The Oxford team can hardly grumble because the press did not print stories that were not made available to them."

This is correct to a point. The problem was, the rules of British science and Florey's sense of appropriate behavior demanded constraint on seeking public attention. However wronged he felt, no part of his character would allow him to call a press conference and point out the achievements of his group. He did, however, try to correct the record. On several occasions Florey privately aired his grievances to those he felt could legitimately plead his case: Mellanby at the MRC and Henry Dale at the Royal Society. Both counseled silent patience.

Florey abided by this stricture and played by the rules, and he resented that others did not. It drove him wild that Fleming basked in the spotlight shone on him by his supporters, and that they were not criticized for grasping more than their due. It was one thing to stay in the shadows when everyone else did; but Florey and his Oxford colleagues felt that if credit was to be given, it should be given to all.

So work at Oxford continued out of public view. In mid-September 1942, two hundred gallons of penicillin broth were sent to Oxford from Kemball, Bishop in milk cans that were acquired for them through the Ministry of Supply. For the next year, there were shipments of 150 gallons to Oxford every ten days. The contributions from Kemball, Bishop and ICI were sufficient to manufacture much of the penicillin for the 187 cases treated by Ethel in 1942 and 1943.

Fleming, too, wanted increased production of penicillin, and he provided some of the impetus for organizing government involvement in its manufacture. After being quiet about penicillin for ten years, now that it was a success, he was suddenly a leading proponent. Shortly before Lambert was discharged from the hospital on September 9, Fleming called his friend Sir Andrew Duncan, the Minister of Supply, to impress on him how valuable penicillin could be. Duncan in turn spoke with Sir Cecil Weir, the director general of Stores and Equipment and therefore the person in charge of medical supplies. (This effort was the "certain thing . . . which may have an important bearing on the large scale production," Fleming mentioned in his letter of September 2.) On September 25, Weir chaired a meeting attended by, among others, Fleming, Florey, and representatives of ICI and the Therapeutic Research Corporation (TRC), a wartime research alliance of five of the largest British major pharmaceutical firms—Boots, British Drug Houses, Glaxo Laboratories, May and Baker, and the Wellcome Foundation; the TRC also shared information with the U.S. Office of Scientific Research and Development and its Committee on Medical Research and Development.

According to the minutes of the meeting, Florey had clear complaints. It was well and good that these firms were sharing information, but he was now out of the information loop. He had given the American companies all the information on penicillin his team had developed, but suddenly the American companies could not share their information with him—it had been declared secret and could only be imparted to the TRC and those who worked with it. The TRC immediately agreed that it would pass to Florey all information from America "without restraint."

While the production of penicillin was more and more under control, publicity about the drug was not. Florey believed that it was premature to make a fuss about penicillin and that the present air of sensationalism was unseemly. A British Broadcasting Company (BBC) program in October so irked him that he fired off a complaint to its director general:

> Did your officers consider whether it was in the public interest to call attention to a substance of therapeutic value which is unprocurable except in minute amounts? And is likely to remain so for a long time to come? This type of publicity, which has been widespread in the press, has resulted in a flood of pathetic letters from as far away as Western Australia and Saskatchewan. . . .
>
> You clearly cannot remedy what has already been broadcast without more publicity which is highly undesirable, but I should like to suggest that, before you let your script-writers loose on scientific subjects which they do not understand, they might at least be instructed to have the courtesy to consult those involved and be told that you place a high value on accuracy and truthfulness.

The joint director general of the BBC responded:

> . . . I have now had an opportunity of looking into the point that you raised.
>
> The script of the short programme on Penicillin was written by Mr. Johnston Abraham, the surgeon, in close consultation with Dr. Alexander Fleming, who provided information on which the broadcast was based and who subsequently read the finished script and agreed to it being broadcast.
>
> We aim at a high standard of accuracy and truthfulness and fully recognize the need, in dealing with scientific subjects, for consultation;

it was felt that in dealing with the story of the discovery of Penicillin we could safely rely on the authoritative guidance of Dr. Fleming.

Florey was not impressed:

It is clear that you took steps to ensure accuracy and truthfulness, except the obvious one of consulting the laboratory in which the research on penicillin is now being carried on. My criticism of inaccuracies on certain points still remains. . . . Dr. Fleming would, I am sure, be aware of these inaccuracies. Possibly your producer's desire for dramatic presentation required more artistic license than is justified in dealing with scientific matter.

These really are points of detail. Had you seen fit to consult me as the person now developing therapeutic use of this medicine, I should, for reasons mentioned in a previous letter, have asked you most sincerely and strongly not to publicise the work at this moment.

Which may well be why the BBC did not ask Florey in the first place.

Florey's ire peaked in December and he sought counsel from Henry Dale, at the time probably the most powerful man in British science.

Dear Sir Henry,

I should be very glad of your advice on the following matter.

As you know, there has been a lot of undesirable publicity in the newspapers and press generally about penicillin. I have taken a firm line here and said there was to be nothing whatever done in the matter of interviews with the press or in any other way. Gardner I know thinks I have been rather wrong about this.

I had a letter from Fleming in which he assured me he was endeavouring to do the same, and I accepted that at its face value and thought that this newspaper publicity would cease. I have now quite good evidence, from the Director-General of the B.B.C. in fact, and also indirectly from some people at St. Mary's, that Fleming is doing his best to see that the whole subject is presented as having been foreseen and worked out by Fleming and that we in this Department just did a few final flourishes. You can see what I mean in the article published in "Britain" to-day, complete with photograph of Fleming and so on.

This steady propaganda seems to be having its effect even on scientific people in that several have now said to us "But I thought you had done something on penicillin too." I am quite aware that anyone who takes the trouble to read the literature can see the facts clearly and this sort of thing of course only arises when, by what now appears to be an extremely fortunate stroke, one has something of rather startling properties.

I would like your advice as to whether the best policy is still to say nothing or, as has been suggested to me, to try to get an article published in *Nature* setting out the matter in some proportion. I would, as I said, have done nothing if it had not become clear that Fleming was not behaving in the best possible manner.

I am sorry to trouble you with this but your mature experience would be of great assistance, as I keep being urged to write something.

Dale's response six days later to "My dear Florey" urged restraint, not because Florey's concerns were unfounded but because Dale felt Florey had important responsibilities beyond claiming his scientific due. Dale was then the president of the Royal Society. Being elected a fellow of the Royal Society and entitled to place the initials F.R.S. after one's name was, and is, a career high point. Usually only one scientist in each of eight disciplines—mathematics, physics, chemistry, engineering sciences, geology, botany, zoology, and physiology and medical sciences— was elected each year. (There are ten categories now.) In later years Florey took pride that his election in 1941 was based almost entirely on work that predated penicillin. Fleming, seventeen years older than Florey, had been put up for membership in 1923, following the publication of his first paper on lysozyme. In that era candidates were considered for five years; after a three-year hiatus, supporters could resubmit their names, which had been done each time for Fleming. Thus going into the nominating meetings of January 1943, Fleming had been considered fourteen times without election. Dale was well aware of this.

I hope I may suggest that you do nothing about an article which anyone could regard as intended to answer, or to correct, any statement made on Fleming's behalf, until we have had the chance of a talk which I should welcome. I should not feel entitled to ask this, if it were not for the fact that you are a member of the R. S. Council, and that in a little over a month from now you will begin to take part in the most difficult and responsible jobs which the Council has to undertake, and in which its function ought to be as clearly above suggestion of partisan feeling or influence as that of a judge. I mean the annual selection of the nominations for the Fellowship, from the list of those who have been put forward by their friends as candidates. Among such candidates is Fleming, and it is within my knowledge that some members of the relevant Committee were very much displeased and dissatisfied because [the Australian Sir Frank] Burnet was last year, in the Committee's final selection, preferred to either of the two other candidates, of whom Fleming was one. [It is not as if Burnet were undeserving of Royal Society fellowship: he would share a 1960 Nobel Prize with Peter Medawar for the discovery of acquired immunological intolerance.] I have little doubt that his claim will be raised again this year, and I am sure that it is important that you should not at this stage, even by publishing what appears to you a completely neutral and unbiased statement of the history of penicillin, give anybody an excuse for suggesting that you are acting against any election which Fleming may have.

I shall welcome a fuller discussion anytime you come to London.

Florey's selection as a council member so quickly after his election as an F.R.S. was a great honor that came with a greater disadvantage. Because the Royal Society conducted its nominations in secret, Florey was duty-bound not to share this letter with his colleagues, who were left to feel that he never pressed their case. Chain was particularly aggrieved that Florey appeared not to fight for the Oxford group's due. In March 1943, Fleming was, indeed, and at last, elected a Fellow of the Royal Society, a deserved honor that added to his luster.

Production of penicillin in England and in the United States was now on two separate courses. Through the beginning of 1943, however, it was still so limited in either country that little or none would be available for civilians in the foreseeable future. Treatment of U.S. soldiers began, in April 1943, on patients from the Pacific war zone with infections that had defied treatment for a year or more: these included compound fractures, soft tissue wounds, and septicemia. By the end of the year, penicillin was the accepted treatment for pus-producing infections and the War Production Board recognized that much more penicillin had to be made as quickly as possible. Abbott Laboratories, Merck, Pfizer, Squibb, and Winthrop Chemical Company—the five American companies that had produced the bulk of penicillin to date—were soon joined by twenty-one other chemical and pharmaceutical firms that were given financial assistance by the WPB. Production skyrocketed.

Penicillin suddenly had all the trappings of a gold rush. Eventually even R. D. Defries at the Connaught Laboratories in Toronto, who dismissed penicillin's possibilities when Florey had visited him in 1941, got his lab to produce it. Ronald Hare, who worked first at St. Mary's and then at Connaught, described the scramble for production in America in *The Birth of Penicillin*. Most of the production was done by large chemical companies, but a few smaller companies also scrambled to cash in.

> One was so successful an adaptation of a plant for the production of mushroom spawn that, for a time, its owner was looked upon as the coming man in the industry. But some were started by amateurs who seemed to be doing it as much for fun as from patriotic or pecuniary motives. One was in a shop in the main street of a little country town with a basement full of inflammable liquids, and was the worst fire trap I have ever seen. . . . But the most remarkable was run by a businessman employing a bacteriological technique entirely his own invention, based mostly on old whisky bottles sterilized by steam direct from a boiler on the point of bursting, in the Stygian gloom of a derelict factory in the meaner part of Brooklyn.

All this effort paid off in a way that could only leave the British envious. In the first five months of 1943, 400 million units of penicillin were produced in America—enough to treat about 180 severe cases; in the following seven months, 20.5 *billion* units were manufactured.

By D-day, June 6, 1944, production was 100 billion units per month—enough for forty thousand cases.

The effort of Newton Richards had much to do with this. He organized, lobbied, and testified often before one congressional group or another in pursuit of funds to expand production. At one of the hearings, a congressman asked, "Doctor, will all these things you are working on tend to lengthen the span of human existence?" The war had been going on for a long time, and, as a friend of Richards put it, "We were all getting to be a bit frazzled."

"God forbid," Richards answered.

The greatest obstacles to the production of penicillin in commercial quantity were the chemical engineering problems of large-scale deep fermentation. For penicillin, this meant finding a strain that could prosper while submerged in the medium; after a couple of enhancements by scientists, the form found on the cantaloupe by "Moldy Mary" Hunt did just that. Then came the challenge of how to distribute sterile air throughout the mixture evenly, which had to be continuously stirred to feed fresh nutrients to the mold.

Scientists at Pfizer were the first to solve these problems. They applied the lessons they had learned in the deep fermentation of the dietary supplement gluconic acid and were willing to take the financial gamble that they could do the same with penicillin.

Penicillin turned out to be much more difficult to work with than gluconic acid, but one by one a dozen technical problems were solved. Sterile air was shot into the tank of broth through a high-pressure nozzle in the bottom of the vessel. To prevent the mold from doing the natural thing of gathering on the surface, where it finds the oxygen it needs to live, a central shaft with blades like those in a washing machine was built into the machine. The resulting violent agitation mixed the oxygen into the broth and allowed the mold to breathe anywhere in the tank; it gave the spores the equivalent of an Aqua-Lung.

Pfizer's effort paid off handsomely: by the end of 1945, the company was making more than half of all the penicillin in the world. Between 1943 and 1945, the price per million units of penicillin—enough to treat one average case—dropped from $200 to $6.

———

To test the effectiveness of penicillin on the battlefield, at the end of May 1943, Florey and Hugh Cairns went to North Africa for three months to oversee the use of penicillin on wounded soldiers. Cairns was an Australian friend and fellow Rhodes scholar who was now a consultant surgeon to the army with the rank of brigadier. They worked on three hundred wounded soldiers in several field hospitals from Algiers to Tripoli to Cairo to answer the two questions they posed: "Can penicillin be used effectively in the field at all?" And, if so, "How much is required and at what place in the army organization can it be used to best advantage?"

It was soon clear that the quicker penicillin was used in the field, the better, but the case of Lieutenant Douglas Carr was an example of its usefulness in the most dire instances.

On April 23, a cannon shell from a Luftwaffe fighter plane had exploded in the open turret of Carr's Royal Armored Corps tank as he and his crew patrolled the Libyan Desert. The shrapnel ripped wounds on both of Carr's arms, his left leg, and around his left eye. He was taken to a field hospital, where six pieces of metal were removed from his right arm and his lacerations were cleaned and dressed. Millions of soldiers in World War I had died from the resulting infection in wounds of this kind.

Within a month Carr was fighting for his life. Weakened by fever and with only a faint heartbeat, he collapsed near midnight on May 26 with a severe pain in his right forearm. Doctors removed the dressing, revealing a pulsating wound. The next day he was transferred to a special field hospital in Tripoli, where penicillin was being tested.

On May 28 and for the next five days, Lieutenant Carr received 2.5 cc's of penicillin, and though he remained weak, he showed improvement. On June 3, however, he began to hemorrhage and collapsed. A blood transfusion restored him, and the next day he was given 4 cc's of penicillin, then 6 cc's on June 5. On June 6, he hemorrhaged twice more and his fever spiked to 103 degrees F (39.4 degrees C).

Surgeons put Carr under general anesthesia and opened the wound in his arm and immediately saw the cause of his infection: a foul-smelling bacteria-laced blood clot that reminded them of a placenta. They cleared away the decayed flesh down to the ligament, swabbed penicillin powder over the surface, sewed the arm back together, and began injections of 3 cc's of penicillin every three hours.

By the next morning Carr's temperature had fallen below normal, his pulse was strong and regular, and his general condition was good. Over the following week, injections continued every three, then four, then six hours as his health was restored. On the morning of June 13, his doctors decided the infection was gone and penicillin treatment was stopped. On June 19, barely three weeks after he was near death, Carr's arm had healed so fully that no further bandages were necessary. A month later, he boarded a troop ship bound for home.

The efficient dispatch of General Rommel's Afrika Corps by the Anglo-American forces led by Field Marshal Bernard Montgomery and General Dwight Eisenhower at first complicated the medical mission. Florey and Cairns intended to treat fresh wounds; instead, they found soldiers like Carr, with festering wounds weeks or months old. This allowed Florey to show penicillin's value as a drug of last resort but did not help him determine its usefulness as a first treatment. War, however, never lacks long for casualties, and the invasion of Sicily that began on July 10 brought the fresh cases they hoped to help. It was soon evident, they later wrote, "that it was far too late to start penicillin treatment weeks or months after wounding, at a Rear Base Hospital, and that it should be tried much earlier, before the establishment of serious infection."

Standard treatment at the time entailed leaving wounds open until some healing was evident; experience had shown that stitching up wounds with debris still in them led to awful infections, including gangrene. Florey and Cairns proposed the medically heretical notion that, instead, wounds should have penicillin powder sprinkled in them (this used less than an injection) and then immediately be sewn shut, leaving a little rubber tube sticking out to allow administration of penicillin solution. When healing was complete, the tube was removed and the hole stitched. As with any new medical procedure, this idea was not immediately embraced; even though the traditional treatment often led to massive infection, doctors were reluctant to discard the most proven course for a speculative one. One day, as Florey demonstrated his technique, an army surgeon looking on was heard to mutter, "It's murder—bloody murder." Florey later wrote: "There is no doubt that even after viewing the wonderful results that penicillin can achieve most surgeons and most administrators, if forced to choose between penicillin and sulphonamides, would say, 'Give us sulphonamides every time.' " But they also won many converts.

While Florey was in North Africa he wrote often to Ethel, who was doing her detailed clinical work with penicillin at the Birmingham Accident Hospital. The letters are chatty and offer a sense of a shared mission. They also are a counterpoint to their often-contentious relationship at home. Perhaps Howard knew that by writing rather than speaking, there could be no misinterpretation due to her deafness, and in this way they could collaborate without argument. In July, he told her:

We are now established in a new place which is hot as hell. We sit all day in a bath of sweat. I drink 9-10 pints a day. The nights are quite good and as we sleep in tents we get what coolness is going. Everyone is most helpful. The only fly in the ointment is to have [Lieutenant Colonel Ian] Fraser about. He talks more nonsense in a confident manner than anyone I have ever encountered. The surgeons we have now working all have much experience of war wounds and are listening to what we say. We have 4 lots of general surgeons and 2 neurological teams working and a certain amount of data is beginning to accumulate. I believe it might be possible to make radical alterations in war surgery if administrative difficulties can be overcome. These are pretty formidable and the optimum conditions may not be possible.

We are using tubes amongst other things for putting in the p. In the first 10 wounds with tubes & 5 days (twice daily) of 250 units p. All appear to be healing. . . . They were dirty to begin with, then excised and sewn up—a thing no-one was doing before.

By August, Florey's news was even better. His impatience with what he considered stupidity was also evident:

Results on the whole are quite impressive. The patients are taking a great interest in their wounds and one chap . . . perfectly healed all while on a bed pan is most upset as he thinks he has let the side down. The nurses are getting keen and find the tube work less arduous than ordinary dressing and they can see how much better the patients are doing. Everyone at this hospital is doing their best—the chief surgeon being one of the most helpful we've come across. I had however a lunch with the consulting orthopaedian who started giving raspberries. He had the outlook associated with orthopaedics. It was a very great advantage not being in the army because I was able to give him a few home truths and I seem to have been in form that day.

Florey and Cairns also showed conclusively that penicillin was highly effective against another common war wound, as he told Ethel:

Ten cases of resistant gonorrhea have been treated with quite dramatic results. They were sulphapyridine [the British-manufactured sulfa drug more commonly known as M&B 693] resistant and appear to have cleared completely in 2 days. We have managed to see a couple of Roman ruins and there is much local color to be observed whenever we emerge from the hospitals.

Everyone is doing their best and working hard. I have lost 10 lbs and am getting a stylish figure again.

Gonorrhea was widespread among British troops in North Africa, particularly so among the more adventurous commandos and paratroopers, and the problem was serious. Several thousand soldiers needed for the invasion of Sicily and the later campaign in Italy were sidelined by the disease, which increasingly did not respond to sulfa drugs. One possible cause of the problem was the French doctors who supervised the Tunis brothels; in many instances, they gave the women small amounts of sulfonamides to mask the disease when they were checked for it, but not enough to prevent its being passed from one customer to the next.

The ten British soldiers cured by penicillin within forty-eight hours—"it was just like turning off a tap," one doctor said—raised a problem of another kind: Should the limited supply be used on the libertines or should it be saved for the inevitable wounded to come? Florey and Cairns were adamant that it should be saved for soldiers whose infections were not self-inflicted, not only because they were concerned how it would look to people back in England, but also because this would allow them to do more research on battle casualties. Major General L. T. Poole, the army's director of pathology, found merit in both opinions and decided not to decide; rather, he sent a query up the line of command, which eventually reached all the way to the prime minister. Churchill was masterful in his nonresponse: "This valuable drug must on no account be wasted. It must be used to the best military advantage." Poole divined that this meant to cure the libertines, who were then able to go into battle. It was a wise choice; the Italian campaign lasted from the beginning of October 1943 through May 1944, and every soldier was needed. By the time wounded soldiers had been given all the British supply of penicillin, the Americans had enough to make up the difference.

Also in the summer of 1943, penicillin was found to be not one thing but at least two: tests showed that British penicillin, produced by surface culture, had a slightly different chemical composition than that in the United States produced by deep fermentation in corn steep liquor. In Britain, the homemade product was called penicillin I and the American, penicillin II; the Americans called theirs penicillin G and Oxford's penicillin F. (In 1944, British scientists found penicillin III and showed it matched one produced at Peoria, called penicillin X.) Scientists at ICI discovered that different strains of mold and different brewing conditions produced different, though closely related, penicillins; they have a common nucleus but differ in the structure of their side chains. All this work provided helpful clues to cracking penicillin's complex chemical code.

At the same time both British and American chemists discovered that the penicillin molecule contained sulfur as well as the already known components of carbon, hydrogen, oxygen, and nitrogen. This rather simple oversight had caused many difficulties in understanding penicillin's chemistry. Taking sulfur into account allowed Abraham, Chain, and others at the Dunn School to postulate that, along with its other special qualities, penicillin had at its base what is called a beta-lactam ring of three carbon atoms and a nitrogen atom, something that had never been found in a naturally occurring product. If Abraham and Chain were right, this anomaly meant that producing synthetic penicillin would be very difficult and very costly.

Robert Robinson, the distinguished chemist at the Dyson Perrins Laboratory up South Parks Road from the Dunn School—he won the 1947 Nobel Prize in chemistry—put forward a competing theory giving penicillin a more conventional chemical structure, which led to some testiness between the two labs. In 1945, X-ray crystallography by Oxford's Dorothy Crowfoot Hodgkin proved Abraham and Chain right; this breakthrough and others like it won her the 1964 Nobel Prize in chemistry. Abraham later developed cephalosporin, the other major beta-lactam antibiotic. By the time of his discovery, the British attitude toward patents had reversed. Abraham patented all chemical variations of cephalosporin and created two trusts for the bulk of the royalties: one for the Dunn School and Lincoln College, the other for the university. So far they have received about £80 million from them.

13

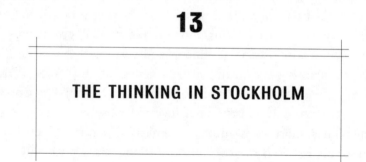

THE THINKING IN STOCKHOLM

From November 29 through December 1, 1943, Roosevelt, Churchill, and Joseph Stalin met in Tehran to plan the Allied strategy against Germany and to consider the postwar political issues. They agreed that Operation Overlord—the invasion of Normandy—would begin in May 1944, and their joint statement at the end of the meeting declared, "We express our determination that our nations shall work together in war and in the peace that will follow."

As Churchill traveled back to London, he became ill with pneumonia in Carthage. His medical treatment there has become the third part of an enduring myth: Alexander Fleming's father saved young Winston Churchill from drowning; in gratitude, Churchill's father paid for Fleming's medical education, which led to the discovery of penicillin; then, in 1943, Churchill was saved from pneumonia by penicillin. None of it is true: no biography of Churchill mentions a near drowning in Scotland; Fleming's education was paid for by the £250 legacy from his uncle and the prizes he won for his academic excellence; Churchill did not receive penicillin in Tunisia. Rather, Churchill's physician Lord Moran summoned to Carthage Dr. Robert Pulvertaft, who was testing on war wounds in Cairo the rather weak penicillin sent him by Florey, to do pathological tests on Churchill's blood. As Pulvertaft wrote to Leonard Bickel, "When I learned that Churchill had pneumonia I suggested to Lord Moran that he should use penicillin, but he had never had experience with its administration, and was quite adamant. . . . [Churchill] was saved by sulphonamides, and fortunately so, because I had no penicillin on hand which I could be sure was non-toxic." The drug Moran administered was M&B 693, made by the British firm May and Baker.

Among their other plans made at Tehran, Churchill, Roosevelt, and Stalin approved a joint American-British scientific trip to Moscow by two scientists from each country to talk about a variety of advances, including penicillin. Florey was asked to represent Britain on the Moscow mission and to join him he picked Gordon Sanders, who, besides his ingenious design of the penicillin manufacturing equipment, had done significant work on blood transfusion at Oxford.

As with the trip to America in 1941, all plans were secret. Florey and Sanders left Oxford for London at two-thirty A.M. on December 23. Before flying out on a military plane on December 24, Sanders wrote in his diary, they went to see "a dreadful American comedy" and the Alexander Korda film *Sahara* ("pretty poor")—though they did like a newsreel of Tarawa in the Gilbert Islands.

Their plane landed in Marrakech, Morocco, at four A.M. Christmas Day. "Merry Christmas," Florey grumbled to Sanders as they walked across the tarmac, but both were cheered after a shower and a breakfast, Sanders wrote, of "all those wonderful things to eat again: Real grapefruit, two fried eggs and two real pork sausages, white bread and good coffee." Christmas dinner, however, was sandwiches in a hot shed in Algiers.

Thirty hours after leaving England, they arrived in Cairo where, Sanders noted, Florey "dealt sharply with an officious man at the British Embassy" who felt that they should be traveling on R.A.F. rather than American planes, one of which had flown them in. After a minute or two of this "lecturette," Florey snapped, "That is not a matter under discussion." On the crowded American plane between Cairo and Tehran, Florey and Sanders perched uncomfortably on hinged aluminum seats, called frying pans because of their shape, and hoped to keep their breakfast down.

"One flies up to 13,000 feet over most ferocious looking mountains," Florey wrote to John Fulton, "and as our pilot remarked, 'You might just as well give your soul to God as your ass belongs to the devil.' "

In Tehran Florey came down with bronchopneumonia, and,

between a short stay in the American army hospital, weather problems, and Russian red tape, it was twenty-seven days before they could travel on. They finally arrived in cold and snowy Moscow in late January and were billeted in the National Hotel, which, Florey told Fulton, was at first quite luxurious.

"Every day the Peruvian and Colombian (I think) diplomats sent a note to [Baird] Hastings [of the American delegation] saying how gratified they were to have in their midst scientists so distinguished that they should assure a hot water supply. However it went cold in 10 days and the lamentable truth appeared that the hot water was due to members of the Supreme Soviet who were staying in the hotel!"

By the time Florey returned to England after ninety-seven days away—seventeen of them traveling and twenty-five waiting for planes—he was exhausted but told Fulton that "I get the greatest pleasure from my association with the Army—I'm now consultant pathologist." However, the pleasures associated with penicillin had eroded away. He wrote to one of his sisters about "the spectacle of everybody who has ever had the slightest bit to do with it crowding in to prove how important their contributions to the matter are." To Fulton he confided, "I'm strenuously trying to get out of the penicillin racket as it seems to arouse all the worst instincts in those who have anything to do with it. The place is full of busybodies and committees but the main thing is that supplies are increasing."

So, continually, was the discrepancy between the credit given Fleming and that given to the group at Oxford. The *News Chronicle* reported on June 3, 1944, that *Time* magazine had opened a fund for Fleming in honor of penicillin because he had not received any money for his work on it. Perhaps mistakenly thinking that Fleming was penniless and languishing in anonymity, a New York businessman had donated $1,000 (£250) to start the fund.

"To hell with all mankind," he wrote in his letter accompanying the check, "when through indifference to the great men who alleviate pain, it permits them either to starve or to die of broken hearts or to pass their last days in acrimonious obscurity." *Time* matched the $1,000, asked for further contributions from readers, and gave Fleming a free lifetime subscription to the magazine. Fleming was clearly the only name the public associated with penicillin.

On June 19, Florey wrote to Mellanby to ask if Mellanby could extricate him from a position that was now intolerable. Florey explained that everyone at Oxford was irritated by what they saw as "the unscrupulous campaign carried on from St. Mary's calmly to credit Fleming with all the work done here. I have sufficient evidence of one sort and another that this is a deliberate and clever campaign." Florey reiterated that even though some of his colleagues urged him to speak out, he had refrained because until now he had been convinced that the matter would "die down and that no one who mattered would be influenced by the Press."

He contrasted his two public lectures given at the invitation of the Royal Institution and the Royal Society of Arts to those of Fleming, who "has been interviewed apparently without cease, photographed, etc. (we have complete 'archives' of this here), with the upshot that he is being put over as the 'discoverer of penicillin' (which is true) with the implication that he did all the work leading to the discovery of its chemotherapeutic properties (which is not true)." The result was that "at most, we 'developed' the subject here.

"You of course know how dishonest this is and might reply 'why worry.' This has been our line and would continue to be if it were not that my colleagues here feel things are going much too far." While no one at Oxford wanted special credit, still people there were "getting quite naturally restive at seeing so much of their work going to glorify and even financially enrich someone else."

Particularly galling was Fleming's election as a member of the New York Academy of Sciences along with Frederick Gowland Hopkins, one of the giants of British science. This was evidence to Florey that scientists whom he had long believed would sort out proper credit instead were blinded by fallacious reporting that Florey saw as more than unenlightened. "During the last week several people—including some nonscientists—have asked me if there wasn't something a bit peculiar about the propaganda, and one of them, who is in a good position to know, lays a good deal of it at Lord Moran's door."

Florey suggested that the Medical Research Council issue a statement to set straight how penicillin was developed. Not only had the MRC supported the work at Oxford, Florey believed that it was the only group able to counter "the Mary's propaganda." Besides, he added pointedly, "The present situation might not have arisen if you had been issuing your regular annual reports," which had been suspended because of wartime shortages. Fair play demanded no less than Mellanby's intervention. All this pleading was not meant to get " 'something for myself,' " he explained. "I have always made it clear how much was due the other workers here."

Then he wrote the most apt description of the whole penicillin saga.

"Nor should anyone suppose that we have performed any great intellectual feats here. All we did was to do some decent experiments and have the luck to hit on a substance with astonishing properties."

It is an evaluation shared by Heatley, who later said: "Apart from the chemistry, which of course was a very difficult subject . . . the work that was done at Oxford was pretty straightforward. There really wasn't anything original in it. It was a question of: here is a product; here is a method of making something. What is the something? How do you make it? How do you extract it? And so on. There was nothing original in any of the work except the chemistry. It was just a question of applying already-known techniques, or perhaps modifying them in different ways, and you're bound to get an answer."

As Henry Harris puts it, without in any way minimizing Florey's accomplishments, "Florey was a practical scientist, not a great one. He was not a seer, a conceptualist. He was no Darwin or Pasteur or Einstein or Ehrlich, and he never thought of himself in that league. Great scientists are volcanoes who turn their science upside down."

Great scientists, he adds, generate the conceptual frameworks for whole fields of study. "Immense tracts of modern physics have readily discernable origins in Newton; before Pasteur and Koch bacteriology as a science can hardly be said to have existed; before Mendel there was no coherent genetics; before Darwin no clear perception of the principles governing the mutability of the living world; before Ehrlich no rational foundation for chemotherapy." No one connected with penicillin fits that bill, even though what was produced affected all of humanity. "But," Harris adds, "Florey had one supreme virtue: he knew exactly what had to be done, and he got it done."

Mellanby's immediate response on June 20 to Florey's appeal

showed no awareness that any story repeated often enough eventually becomes the conventional wisdom. Yes, the Oxford group was in "a difficult position . . . owing to the unusual attitude Fleming has taken up in response to the public acclamation of penicillin," but Florey's reticence was "above criticism" and "the most desirable" path.

> You need have no doubt whatever in your mind that scientific men, in this country at least, and doubtless most of them in other countries, have appraised the situation correctly and know that, from the point of view of scientific merit, your work and that of your colleagues stands on a much higher level than that of Fleming.
>
> I realize how irritating your position must be, if you are at all affected by what appears in the popular press, but you can be quite certain that this is an ephemeral reaction which means little or nothing, and the only appreciation which is worth bothering about is that of your scientific peers. In time, even the public will realize that . . . the thing that has mattered most has been the persistent and highly meritorious work of your laboratory. The dish you have turned out is so good that you must swallow the rather nauseating but temporary publicity ingredient with a smile.

That was easy enough for Mellanby to say, but it has proved fanciful: more than sixty years after the work at Oxford, it is Fleming's name that most people recall when they think of penicillin.

Florey was right in thinking that Moran was involved with the "propaganda" from St. Mary's, but Moran's interest was not so much in getting undue credit for Fleming at the expense of Florey as it was to use that credit to ensure the hospital's survival. Moran had already once saved St. Mary's Medical School, after the University Grants Committee had deemed early in his tenure as dean in the 1920s that the school was unsuitable for its purpose. Moran was keenly aware that, after the war, medicine would forever change and therefore, inevitably, so would hospitals. He was eager to help St. Mary's and the Inoculation Department adapt to these changes. On August 10, 1944, he wrote to Anthony de Rothschild, the chairman of St. Mary's.

I gather that it is proposed to precede the hospital appeal by a special penicillin appeal for the Inoculation Department. I confess that I view this procedure with some misgiving. It is true that an appeal by St. Mary's at the present time must depend for its success largely on Fleming's work and that therefore his wishes ought to be most carefully considered, and it is also true that the discovery of penicillin may affect the sale of vaccines. Nevertheless I see no future for any teaching hospital that has not six hundred beds. There are too many medical schools in London and the authorities would not be sorry if some of them dropped out. . . . I think ultimately, taking long views, it would be little advantage to the Inoculation Department to have invested funds and endowments if anything happened to the school. . . . I have opportunities of learning the policy of the Government and of those concerned with education which have led me to believe that I ought to put before you, as Chairman, the vital importance of bringing the beds up to six hundred.

Fleming was involved with this as well. On August 15, de Rothschild answered Moran. Part of his letter refers to the downside for hospitals after penicillin—almost no one now needed the kind of care the septic wards offered, and as they were shut down, so, too, did a stream of revenue dry up.

I feel sure that all connected with the Inoculation Department fully appreciate the importance of [the] loss of income owing to the invention of penicillin. We discussed the matter especially from the point of view of St. Mary's Hospital and I had the advantage and support of Sir Alexander Fleming. After thorough examination of the question I felt that there was no alternative but to accept their decision to make a penicillin appeal in the near future. They thought that this appeal could be limited to a comparatively narrow circle of interested parties who would be likely to give large subscriptions, including certain Trusts or Companies who might be less disposed to give directly to the hospital. They promised to endow a certain number of beds in the Hospital, according to the amount they raised, and they further agreed that their appeal should not last in any event longer than the end of this year; they also pointed out that there was nothing whatever to prevent the

Hospital making use of its association with the invention of penicillin when it launched its own appeal and that in fact by that time penicillin would have brought relief to a very much larger circle of patients, so that the delay might even have some compensating advantages.

In the King's Honors List in June 1944, Fleming and Florey were each made a Knights Bachelor. Fleming's name was in the lead in the report in the *Times*: "His Majesty the King held an investiture at Buckingham Palace and conferred the honour of knighthood on thirty-eight gentlemen. Among those who received the accolade was Professor Alexander Fleming." In most stories about the event, Florey's name generally was found in the small type used for lists.

When Fleming returned to St. Mary's following the investiture that for safety was conducted in the basement of Buckingham Palace, Almroth Wright's daily afternoon tea was under way in the library. Wright made no comment when Fleming entered the room and no one spoke for two or three minutes. Jealousy overcame the old man, whose lifelong conviction that vaccines were the best answer to disease had been at least in part disproved by his protégé's accomplishment. Wright turned his back on Fleming and launched into a harangue that chemotherapy would be the ruin of genuine research—this after he had so publicly awarded Fleming the laurel wreath of victory for his discovery of penicillin.

Wright, however, was about the only person to turn his back on Fleming. Unmentioned in all the letters and discussions between Florey, Mellanby, and Dale, but impossible not to be on everyone's mind, was the greatest recognition of all, the Nobel Prize. The prizes had been suspended in 1940 (there also was no 1939 Peace Prize) because of the war, and, in 1944, there was first a rumor and then an official announcement that in October they would be reinstated retroactively to 1943. The opinion of scientists in countries other than Britain mattered very much in the judging of these prizes, and, if the New York Academy of Sciences had been unable to see that the work at Oxford stood "on a much higher level than Fleming," then what were members of the Nobel Committee in Stockholm thinking in their secret deliberations?

Many in the scientific community were asking themselves precisely that, perhaps none more than John Fulton. In early October, he wrote to Dr. Per J. Hedenius at the Swedish Legation in New York:

> I learned yesterday from a friend who had just flown from England that the British press has published a rumour that Fleming, and Fleming alone, is to be recognized for the discovery of penicillin. I sincerely and most earnestly hope that this is only a rumour. Informed opinion in this country would look upon an award to Fleming alone as most unfortunate and in almost complete disregard for credit where it is really due. Howard Florey and his resourceful team at Oxford are responsible for devising a procedure for the successful extraction of penicillin; they are responsible for proving its clinical usefulness, its mode of assay, its dosage, and the means of its excretion from the body. All this ten years after Fleming had abandoned study of penicillin in the belief that it was too "labile" for clinical use. . . .
>
> It is probably wholly unnecessary for me to mention these things since I have the utmost regard for the critical acumen of the Nobel Committee and especially for the wise guidance [Dr. Göran] Liljestrand has so long given. But if the rumour comes to me as correct, I can only attribute it to the fact that in considerable measure the Committee has been cut off from the facts in the case and that it has been unduly influenced by the Beaverbrook rather than by the medical press of England.
>
> I propose to send no message to Liljestrand, but if you think it worth while to pass on to him the context of this expression of opinion, I shall be glad to have you do so. It represents the considered opinion of a large group in this country including the Division of Medical Sciences of the National Research Council and the officers of the American Medical Association.
>
> P.S. Our recommendation would be, in order of preference:
> Florey alone
> Florey and Chain
> Florey, Chain and Fleming

The rumor became more specific ten days later. On October 17, a headline in the *Daily Mail* announced "Nobel Prize for Fleming of

Penicillin." The story turned out to be only a continuation of the rumor, with the added speculation that because the £8,500 prize had not been awarded since 1939, "some of the accumulated funds may be used to reward Sir Alexander's close collaborator, Professor H. W. Florey, who was knighted with Sir Alexander for his part in the discovery."

Florey, of course, was not Fleming's close or even distant collaborator, but yet another die for a medal of credit had been cast.

Chain was equally worried. Edward Abraham watched as he "became agitated by thoughts that a Nobel Prize would be awarded for penicillin and he would not be among the recipients. He voiced these thoughts to me on several occasions and asked whether he should not take steps to make his contribution more widely known. I advised him to do nothing, but doubted whether he was convinced that this course was best."

If indeed Fleming had Lord Beaverbrook and his newspapers as his press agents, Florey and Chain had a worthy champion in Fulton. Two weeks after his letter to Hedenius, Fulton sent a cable to Liljestrand:

PROFOUNDLY DISTURBED OVER PERSISTENT REPORTS THROUGH BEAVER-BROOK PRESS CONCERNING FLEMING SINCERELY HOPE RUMOUR IS UNFOUNDED SINCE CREDIT FOR ALL CLINICAL DEVELOPMENT BELONGS TO FLOREY AND ASSOCIATES

A few days after Fulton's cable, the Nobel Prizes for physiology or medicine were awarded for 1943 to Henrik Dam and Edward A. Doisy for work on vitamin K, and for 1944 to Joseph Erlanger and Herbert S. Gasser for work on nerve fibers. Fulton immediately wrote to Liljestrand and once again pressed Florey's claim.

We are all much relieved that old Beaverbrook did not sway your committee in the direction of giving the penicillin award to a single person; for had it not been for the imagination, determination, and conviction of Florey and his resourceful team at Oxford, penicillin might never have been heard of as a chemotherapeutic agent. The dramatic part is that the whole development was based on well-conceived animal experimentation. The lack of toxicity was thoroughly established in a great variety of animals before the substance was subjected to clinical trial. . . .

Some of those who heard Florey's story here in July 1941 thought he was crazy. . . . All those, however, who took the trouble to examine his *experimental* evidence in animals realized that he had something possessing great potentialities. . . . There are some in Britain who feel that Fleming should receive full credit for the discovery of penicillin. He made a good observation and wrote an important paper in 1929, but by 1932 he had abandoned all thought of further work on penicillin in the belief that it was too unstable to lend itself to clinical use.

As you are aware, knowledge of the existence of antibiotics goes back to Pasteur; and many, including Fleming, DuBos, and others had envisaged the possibility of putting them to clinical use. But, as with [William] Morton and the introduction of surgical anesthesia, it was Florey who actually did the convincing and effective work and, again as with Morton, it was Florey who took personal responsibility for the first clinical administration of the new agent. There are many in this country and in Britain (I should think the vast majority of informed opinion) who, knowing these facts, share the view that Florey deserves primary credit for the introduction of penicillin. Dr. Fishbein, the editor of the *Journal of the American Medical Association*, is emphatically of this point of view, as you will see from the editorial of 16 September, and it is also shared by Weed and Ross Harrison.

The question of who deserves credit for penicillin echoes the debate over who among Carl Wilhelm Scheele, Joseph Priestley, and Antoine Lavoisier most deserves credit for the discovery of oxygen, which launched the chemical revolution in the late eighteenth century. All three can be said to have "discovered" it, but just what did they discover? Should credit go to Scheele, the first person to make oxygen but who did not publish his findings? Or to Joseph Priestley, who was the first to publish but like Scheele did not understand what he had found? Or to Lavoisier, who was the first to comprehend the value of oxygen as a chemical, gave no credit to the work of Scheele and Priestley, and for more than two hundred years has been considered the father of the chemical revolution?

A particular concern of Fulton's was that because the war limited the dissemination of so much scientific information, the Nobel assessors in Sweden did not have the benefit of knowing the whole story. This seems likely to have been the case, but, even so, he did not need to be quite so worried. Liljestrand and his committee had been considering Fleming, Chain, and Florey jointly since April 1943 but, as Liljestrand wrote to his colleagues, with caution:

> It is clear that penicillin will attract much interest. Very possibly it will prove to be a great chemotherapeutic success but it may be too early to make a judgment as to how reliable it will be. Perhaps it is better to wait and see what the examinations from other directions are because it has been tested over only a small time. . . .
>
> It is likely to show chemotherapeutic success but reliable judgment is not yet there. Therefore I recommend we not to take up Fleming's and Florey's work for penicillin for examination by the Committee.

In England that same spring, there was much interest by two people in a very personal matter. In May 1944, Norman Heatley asked a young woman he fancied to a dance at Oxford. She was unable to go but suggested he instead take a friend of hers, Mercy Bing, a lively and attractive medical student at Somerville College. He did and, to his pleasure, found her a "very agreeable and a very interesting talker. Also amusing and witty." He was particularly taken by Mercy's recounting of a trip to London during which her suitcase "had done a 'projectile vomit' onto the platform. I can't imagine many girls using such language." Mercy, in turn, was impressed by his kindness when, the day following the dance, she developed quite a severe toothache. "I don't know how Norman knew about this, but he appeared with oil of cloves. I was immensely touched and that was really the beginning of my interest." They were married that December. Mercy received her degree in medicine and went on to become a psychologist and the mother of their five children. Sixty years later, she remains the determined, plainspoken, and charming person he fell in love with.

Their courtship coincided with D-day, the Allied invasion of Normandy, on June 6. Almost three years to the day that Florey and

Heatley arrived in New York, American production of penicillin had risen from 0 to 100 billion units per month, enough to treat every Allied casualty. The amount would continue to grow exponentially: By 1951, 25 to 30 trillion units a month were produced; by 1978, the amount was 384.5 trillion units a month.

Also, by summer 1944, there was an emerging consensus regarding the Nobel Prize. "A lot of literature has come from American magazines," Liljestrand wrote in a July 20 memo. The "opinion of many scientists" was that the work of Fleming, Chain, and Florey "opened up a new field in medicine, which appears will result in untold benefits to mankind." He agreed with the many scientists: "Really, very few medical discoveries can be compared to penicillin. . . . It seems obvious that bringing penicillin into therapy is a Nobel Prize winning effort." The question was, who should be awarded the prize—the maximum that can share it is three—and should the money be shared equally?

"Of the three proposed," Liljestrand continued, "Fleming has made the primary discovery. His prize worthiness seems unbeatable to me. . . . Just as clear is that the leaders of the Oxford group are prize worthy because without their work the discovery would have been ignored. . . . Although numerous collaborators helped, it is clear that Chain and Florey are the leaders and should be considered for the prize as well," and he recommended that "the division of the eventual prize" be half for Fleming and half for Chain and Florey.

A month later committee member Nanna Svartz agreed that Chain and Florey were the leaders of the group that did the work and that it was "indisputable" that they "should be honored now that penicillin is available." But, she concluded, "their work is not of the same high class as Fleming's" and she, too, proposed half to Fleming, the other half divided between Chain and Florey.

Perhaps it was a good thing after all that Fulton was so active on Florey and Chain's behalf.

In December 1944, Paquita and Charles returned to England, four and a half years after they left Oxford. Howard stopped in New Haven to pick them up on his way home from a tour of Australia. In the months before they left, the Fultons had several wooden crates built in the basement for them to put in things they wanted to take back. There were also trunks filled with new clothes; Lucia sent more for years to come.

The ten-day trip as part of a convoy of more than fifty hastily constructed Liberty Ships made for a relaxed reunion. Paquita was put in a cabin with several other girls; Charles and Howard were jammed together in a cabin of six men. They passed much of the time playing poker dice on the cabin floor. There were still a few Nazi submarines in the Atlantic. No longer the scourge of the sea-lanes, they now were impotent. Destroyers wove through the convoy and sank six.

"When we got home," Charles says, "Ma was a stranger."

While the children were in America, Ethel devoted all her time to treating patients with penicillin. Paquita feels that "she found it hard to be in the shadow of Pa. Penicillin was her second chance at making a medical difference but she did not make it on her own. She wanted to establish her independent value." Ethel continued to work at full speed after they returned, but, Charles recalls, "She was a very loving mother and she spent a lot of time with us. I think she compensated for the absence of my father, in fact."

Florey returned to find that Fleming's credit for penicillin was greater than ever. By the summer of 1945, he had come to the point at which he felt there was little to do but hope time would eventually allow the Oxford workers the credit they deserved.

"There is a lot of axe grinding going on at present in England," he wrote to Fulton in June, "a frightful campaign emerging from St. Mary's trying to collect money. Oxford has been completely eliminated from the picture as far as the lay public is concerned. These probably don't matter very much but I know that many scientific people here are somewhat annoyed at the general line Fleming and his hospital are pursuing."

A letter from Fulton that August referred to a U.S. visit by Fleming; in June 1945, he received honorary doctorates from Princeton University, the University of Pennsylvania, and Harvard University (having in May been made an Honorary Freeman and Liveryman of the Dyers' Company of the City of London and an Honorary Freeman of the Borough of Paddington).

Fulton had been asked to write an article on antibiotics for *The Atlantic Monthly*, and, he wrote Florey after hearing Fleming speak in New Haven, "I was more than ever eager to write the article, since then there has been an ever mounting emphasis in the local press on the importance of 'F' 's contribution, and the adroit Scot has talked our drug house people out of eighty thousand dollars for St. Mary's. I cannot think how their memories could be so short."

Florey, who handed penicillin to the U.S. drug companies, was denied not only his kilo of penicillin but any acknowledgment or reward from them as well.

"You are a very good friend indeed to get worried over these things," Florey wrote to Fulton in return.

> We are all trying to cultivate the philosophical color associated with Oxford. All one can say is that it comes as a revelation how really unscrupulous one's colleagues—used in a wide sense—can be. 'F' no doubt will get full credit for that one of these days. Since returning he has been to France to the academy of medicine—heavily honored in the papers and neatly woven into the collection of money for Mary's. I have a most interesting exhibit sent to me in connection with the Mary's appeal.

The "exhibit" was an invitation from Paramount Pictures to a July 12, 1945, screening of *The Affairs of Susan*, starring Joan Fontaine, part of a drive to raise £2 million to renovate St. Mary's. It began:

> Dear Sir Howard,
> You will know of the discovery by Professor Sir Alexander Fleming of Penicillin and of the many lives it has saved during the war. You may not, however, be aware that this wonderful discovery was made in the research Department of St. Mary's Hospital, Paddington.

Florey framed the letter and put it in the front hall of the Dunn School. "It seems to cause some visitors great amusement," he wrote to Fulton.

Lord Moran made an appeal on the radio for the hospital. Florey missed the broadcast and asked for a copy of his remarks, "as we have a most interesting collection of articles and such like gathered from the world press."

Moran sent them, along with a note saying, "My 'good cause' appeal was a 4½ minute business designed to bring in the boodle to St. Mary's."

To Fleming's credit, he sometimes made a point of mentioning the work in Oxford. In a speech in Paris on September 7, 1945, he reminded his listeners, "I have had many compliments paid to me regarding penicillin. I want to say again that I only started that story. My compatriots, Raistrick in London, and Florey, Chain, and their coworkers at Oxford carried it on and then large numbers of workers, academic and industrial, in Britain and especially in the United States have made penicillin what it is today."

Few seemed to hear him, then and in the years to come. He was too appealing a character. His shyness, his plain appearance, and his humility—what might have been drawbacks in others—were endearing in Fleming. It wasn't his fault that the world wanted to lionize him; and when the world clamors to lionize you, it is the rarest of persons who tells the world to go away.

In Stockholm that summer and fall, the decision on the Nobel was weighed. One of the many letters of nomination that year was from Henry Dale.

My dear Liljestrand,

I am sending herewith a proposal of my own, for the award of the Nobel Prize for Physiology and Medicine for 1945 to Fleming and Florey, for the discovery of penicillin and its therapeutic applications. It is rather a remarkable story:

There can be no doubt that Fleming made the original discovery, and even a move, though not a very vigorous or determined one, to getting its practical application tried. Nothing came of it, and I think that it is quite certain that we should not have heard anything more about Penicillin and its properties unless Florey, or failing him, somebody else later, and perhaps not yet, had taken up the matter again and pushed the investigation ahead, with a clear recognition of its potential importance, which amounted in itself to something like a rediscovery.

You will have had cases more or less analogous to consider earlier. I am quite sure that, if the committee find it possible to give this recognition this year, and to give it jointly to Fleming and Florey, they will be acting in accordance with the judgment and wishes of all who have been behind the scenes, and have had an opportunity of knowing intimately the nature of the discovery, and the relation of the work of each of the men concerned to that of the other.

As part of the deliberations, Sven Hellerström conducted investigations into the dermatological and venereal values of penicillin and agreed on the choices of Fleming, Florey, and Chain. Evaluator Anders Kristensen wrote, "From this discovery other antibiotics should follow. We don't need any more information to prove Fleming, Florey and Chain should receive the award, although more supplementary information could be gotten. Penicillin is an antibiotic of highest therapeutic value. . . . The 1945 prize should be given to Fleming for the discovery of penicillin and Florey and Chain for its development."

In a letter to his colleagues, Liljestrand noted, "This year even more scientists have recommend Fleming, Florey and Chain—13 of 16 that came in—but only three mention Fleming alone." He also pointed out that there had been a suggestion by an American scientist in Philadelphia for an alternate division of the prize: Fleming and Florey as well as Newton Richards, who "assisted materially in developing its production." But Liljestrand pointed out that Richards's work on production, while valuable, was not a discovery of any kind and therefore not eligible under the Nobel guidelines.

Liljestrand's summary of the other nominations gives a glimpse into the promotion of national favorites. The Belgian scientist André Gratia, who had observed penicillin's effect before Fleming but not followed up on it, suggested the award should be divided equally between Fleming and Florey. Gratia himself was proposed because of his work on antibiotics, but, as Liljestrand pointed out, he had many collaborators and "brought no new meaning. The Belgians just want him there," and the committee should "not take away from Fleming and Florey" by considering him.

On October 25, 1945, Florey, Fleming, and Chain received almost identical telegrams from Hilding Bergstrand in Stockholm. Florey's read:

THE CAROLINE INSTITUTE HAS DECIDED TO AWARD THIS YEARS NOBEL PRIZE FOR PHYSIOLOGY AND MEDICINE TO YOU DOCTOR CHAIN AND PROFESSOR FLEMING JOINTLY FOR THE DISCOVERY OF PENICILLIN AND ITS CURATIVE ACTION IN VARIOUS INFECTIOUS DISEASES

The emphasis by Dale and others on the work seems to have influenced the judges in how the honor should be apportioned. Rather than single out the contribution of one as being more important than the others, the award and prize money were split evenly—one-third to each.

Chain, staying with a friend in New York when he received the news, paced the floor and kept asking, "Is it true? Are you sure?" In an interview in the *New York Times* he praised the British and U.S. pharmaceutical companies for their fast work on the drug but added, "Nobody in our group has received a ha'penny out of this but firms are making millions of dollars—$20,000,000 I heard recently. . . . Our part, of course, was considerably smaller that that of the soldier who fought, but on the other hand, I don't see why a commercial development should get so much money. I thought that the Governments would take over the production of penicillin and there would be no great profits."

The next day John Fulton sent four cables. To Liljestrand he wrote:

NOBEL AWARD BRINGS DEEP SATISFACTION TO ALL FAMILIAR WITH HISTORY OF PENICILLIN

To Chain:

WARMEST CONGRATULATIONS FROM ALL YOUR MANY FRIENDS AT YALE

To Florey:

> ALL IS WELL THAT ENDS WELL. WARMEST CONGRATULATIONS TO YOU ETHEL
> AND ALL MEMBERS OF THE TEAM

The fourth was to the *New York Times* and began,

> CORRECTION IMPERATIVE

The headline announcing the prize read: FLEMING AND TWO CO-WORKERS GET NOBEL AWARD FOR PENICILLIN BOON. The implication (corrected in an editorial the next day) was that Florey and Chain were junior assistants of Fleming. Fulton set the record straight.

> FLOREY AND CHAIN TOOK UP STUDY . . . QUITE INDEPENDENTLY OF FLEMING
> AND WERE IN NO SENSE HIS COWORKERS. FLOREY AND CHAIN ARE RESPONSI-
> BLE FOR DISCOVERING THE THERAPEUTIC POTENTIALITIES OF PENICILLIN AND
> FOR MAKING IT AVAILABLE FOR CLINICAL USE

Even though Florey and Chain now had the prize, they still did not quite have the proper credit. Heatley had none at all.

14

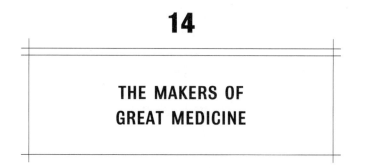

THE MAKERS OF
GREAT MEDICINE

The Nobel Prize awards and ceremonies were the first since the start of the war, and the celebrations surrounding them were an added pleasure after so many years of fighting and privation. Chain wrote to Perrin Long in Washington, D.C., that the "festivities . . . put a considerable strain on my oxidative system, greater even than those imposed by American dinner parties."

Ethel went to Stockholm with Howard ("I had the week of my life," she wrote to Lucia Fulton) and then traveled on to Edinburgh to have an operation that she hoped would improve her hearing. (It did not.) It meant she would miss being with her children for their first Christmas at home in five years, but she felt it was important that she lose no more time from the clinical trials of penicillin she was still conducting.

"I just had a third of my head shaved and am wondering how on earth long it will be before I look presentable again," she continued to Lucia.

I am to have an operation on my ear which according to the surgeon gives me a 60–40 per cent chance of having my hearing restored within normal limits. (Trying not to think of being amongst 35–40% who have bad luck.)

This seems a strange contrast to what I was doing at this time last week—dining in the King's Palace with the Prime Minister and Prince

Berthie for my next door neighbours. We had an absolutely terrific time. People entertained us the whole time we were there and we never got to bed before 2 a.m. . . . . You would have thought it comic to see me at the civic banquet with the Crown Prince and Prince Berthie on either side with all their magnificent decorations and the Crown Princess and aristocracy in their magnificent evening gowns and jewels while poor little me sat there in a 12 year old evening dress and no jewelry but a necklace of pearls Paq lent me! Flos said "Never mind, they'll only say, 'Well she's only a poor scientist. . . .' "

Fleming's refrain was repeated on every occasion—"How I discovered lysozyme and why I did not carry on with penicillin." Chain talked about the cruelest tyranny the world has ever seen which had just ended and about his own race being the most cruelly persecuted on earth— which rather irritated the Swedes. And Flos talked about the threat to freedom of thought and work of scientists that some statesmen and politicians seemed to envision. The *Daily Mail* correspondent was delighted and reported that Flos said "Scientists should rule the world." So there were leaders in the English papers who had taken no notice of the festivities before, saying that this just went to show that scientists should be kept in their place!

Howard enjoyed himself as well, he told John Fulton. "The Swedes really did us proud—one could easily get the impression of being a great man." But parts of the event left him furious.

Dinner next night at the Palace and the King remarking "So it was all an accident" to Chain, Fleming and myself. When he passed on I remarked that he didn't seem the only one that thought that. . . .

The only flaw really was having Fleming about. I refuse to speak to that fellow and he's now annoyed my wife. I'm really mad now about the downright dishonesty with which he presses his way and I hope in time to catch up with him. I'm hoping to write my memoirs for consumption in later years—I am now driven to the conclusion there are extremely few honest people and those who manipulate our destinies are often the shadiest types and capable of the meanest tricks.

After returning from Stockholm my wife went to Edinburgh and had a hole bored in her ear.

Florey never wrote his memoirs. If he had, he might well have claimed that the first beneficiary of penicillin was not Anne Miller or any of the four early cases at Oxford but actually Alexander Fleming. Maxwell Cowan, the pathfinding neuroscientist, makes the point that "Fleming was the first person Florey saved. Without Florey's work he would have gone down as a somewhat eccentric microbiologist."

The Nobel did nothing to repair Chain and Florey's broken relationship, which was exacerbated even more over the publication of *Antibiotics*, the two-volume work that grew from the idea that the pair would write a monograph on the development of penicillin. Chain worried that including chapters written by almost every member of the team would give the impression that his contribution was less than he believed it to be; Florey countered that Chain sought credit for work he did not do. Chain wrote a long letter objecting to particular points in the book after its publication in 1949, but, in most areas, it is the one account of the penicillin story on which all the Oxford parties agree.

The Nobel did allow Chain a forum to argue for a state-owned penicillin factory that would produce the drug more efficiently and cheaper than private firms and to make the case for patents. In this he found a more sympathetic ear than in 1941. His prediction that Britain would have to pay royalties on penicillin proved correct. An added insult was that Andrew Moyer, Heatley's colleague in Peoria, won British patents for his method of production. Although as a U.S. government employee he was prohibited from seeking a patent on his work in the United States, there was no such prohibition for other countries. There was a loud outcry of indignation in England when it became clear that the financial reward for a substance developed in Britain would accrue in the United States. Suddenly, patenting was seen in a new light. Eventually the British National Research Development Corporation was formed to receive the patents on inventions by academics and to oversee their protection and their development. But it is unlikely that either Fleming or Florey and his group would have had much of a claim under any circumstances.

"It is often said in the press here that they got the penicillin out at Oxford and the Americans pinched it," Henry Harris says. "But any British patents wouldn't have lasted long. Fleming's paper put it in the public domain. Patent law was more restrictive at the time. There were only two kinds of patent: One for a new product, and Fleming had already described that in his 1929 paper; and another for a new process. It's doubtful if a commercial product could have been made from surface culture penicillin. Three dimensions were needed, and the Americans already had patents for growing fungi in corn steep in 3-D."

There is also the matter of different penicillins. As Harris points out,

> All the penicillin at Oxford had the structure called penicillin F. Americans were not satisfied with the yield and sought strains with a higher yield. Cantaloupe gave them penicillin G. The question is, do side chains count or just the basic chemical structure? The patent on F would have lasted just a year. When cephalosporin came along, Abraham patented the whole cephalosporin ring. With penicillin, if Abraham had got on to the B-lactam ring earlier, they could have patented that. The idea that the Americans pinched it from the British is twaddle. It was a different mold, a different product.

There was, as well, a vast cultural difference between the ethos of research in Oxford and in the United States. Oxford prized the amateur; the United States was more businesslike. The true scientist-entrepreneurs were the Germans. After Ehrlich, they patented everything.

In 1947, at the request of the British Council, Chain went to Italy to give several lectures on penicillin. His ideas for continuing research and production so changed the thinking of scientists and government officials, including the prime minister, that he was invited to organize and direct a research center for chemical microbiology and a pilot penicillin plant at the Instituto Superiore di Sanitá. He left the Dunn School in the summer of 1948 but did not resign his post. After he arrived in Rome, he wrote to Florey:

> My Dear Professor,
> To my regret I could not say goodbye to you personally as you were in London on the day of my departure. So I have to do it by letter.

I am very sorry that our personal relationship has deteriorated so much during the last years; I think the reason for it is mainly the general imperfection of human nature. I have always deeply regretted this development and I hope that as time goes on the unpleasant episodes—which, after all, were not frightfully important when looked at from a broad viewpoint—may gradually sink into oblivion and we shall remember only the exciting and unique events of the time of our collaboration which a curious fate has destined us to experience together.

A year later, he wrote on the occasion of resigning his post at the Dunn School, to which he did not return for thirty years:

. . . an episode in my life has come to an end which has been rich in elating emotions such as very few people are privileged to experience.

I shall remember with great pleasure, and always with gratitude, the first years of our association in which the foundation for the subsequent work was laid, and I shall try to forget the bitter experiences of the later years which I am sure will sink into insignificance as time goes on.

There is no copy of Florey's reply to Chain's first letter; to the second he wrote:

I hope that your position in Rome will give you all the scope that you need to carry on your work. We shall all follow your progress with interest and hope you will make a great success of your Institute. I only trust that the difficulties of running laboratories will not disillusion you too soon, but I am sure it is best that you should run your own show.

Also in 1949, Chain was finally elected a fellow of the Royal Society. Florey first nominated him in 1944. As with Fleming, membership was elusive, but also as with Fleming (though not to the same extent) he received a large number of honorary degrees and memberships in learned societies. In 1961, he was made Professor of Biochemistry at Imperial College, London, but did not move there until 1964, when he gave up his position in Rome. In 1969, he was knighted.

Chain's ability as a chemical engineer and his understanding of business made him a sought-after consultant to many pharmaceutical companies. He also was a valuable supporter of the Weizmann Institute in Rehovot, Israel, and became a member of its board of governors and later one of the Executive Committee. Chain's commitment to the State of Israel and to Judaism increased as his life went on. He was a generous patron of London's Central Synagogue and donated many of the honoraria he received for lectures and other work.

In 1971, Chain built a home in County Mayo, Ireland, and moved in his Steinway grand piano. He maintained an office at Imperial College for the many consulting projects he undertook, even during a year of poor health that began in 1978. He died in Ireland during his summer holiday in 1979. He was seventy-three.

After the Nobel, Fleming's popularity soared. Over the next ten years he averaged more than one tribute a month, in cities around the globe. He was awarded more than a score of honorary doctorates, was made the Lord Rector of Edinburgh University, received more than fifty medals, prizes, and decorations, and was welcomed as an honorary member of nearly ninety venerable organizations, mostly professional groups such as the Royal Society of New Zealand or the College of Surgeons in Brazil, but other groups saluted him as well. In 1949, he was made an honorary member of the Kiowa Tribe in America and given the name Chief Doy-Gei-Taun—Maker of Great Medicine.

Gwyn Macfarlane argues that Fleming achieved such fame because he was the perfect antihero. After World War II, "ordinary people were sick of dictators, politicians and military leaders and they feared the scientists who could bring themselves to make atom bombs and poison gases. All the self-important characters had brought death and destruction. What greater contrast could there have been in Fleming? . . . When they actually saw, not a dominating, alarming figure, but a simple, modest little man, they went wild with gratitude and affection. When Fleming proclaimed that his discovery of penicillin was an accident, they did not believe him. They were sure that he had worked it all out, but was simply too modest to admit his true genius."

Fleming's wife, Sareen, died in 1949, and in 1953, he married Dr.

Amalia Voureka, a Greek physician's daughter forty-two years his junior, who had come to work in his lab in 1946. An outspoken opponent of totalitarianism, she was particularly active against the junta that came to power in Greece in the 1960s.

On March 11, 1955, Fleming, then seventy-three, died in London from a massive blood clot in his heart. The world mourned. His ashes were interred in the crypt of St. Paul's Cathedral, in the company of two hundred British heroes, including Lord Nelson, the Duke of Wellington, and Christopher Wren, the cathedral's architect.

Among the many proposed memorials—statues, plaques, and buildings named for him, including the Department of Health and Social Security in London—a group organized the Fleming Memorial Penicillin Fund and enlisted Prince Philip, the Duke of Edinburgh, as its patron. This nomenclature did not sit well with the group at Oxford, who complained that it ignored any contribution by them.

There were many Fleming constituencies, including the staff and board of St. Mary's Hospital and the general population of Scotland, but seemingly only one with an interest in the work at Oxford. The problem facing the Oxford group was how to become a recipient of some of the research money that would flow from the memorial without sacrificing the notion that they might have had something of a hand in the development of penicillin. In December 1955, Florey, Gardner, Abraham, Heatley, Jennings, and Sanders met at the Dunn School to hear Florey's report of the negotiations.

"The ball has been passed to us to put straight. I cannot make it any more precise," he told them. "Everyone was peevish. They would do their best to keep the Mary's people under control. If the whole thing was called off they thought Mary's might take [the memorial fund] on even if the Duke did not."

The current thinking, Florey continued, was, "Everyone was fairly clear that they wanted to pass it to a committee nominated by the president of the Royal Society and that committee should have the disposal of the money," but he "was shocked to find" that one of the prime movers of the memorial was "talking of giving out money to all sorts of institutions but nothing to Oxford." This, however, seemed a minority opinion and so Florey "did not point [Oxford's omission]

out. Everyone was full of good will; I think there would be no difficulty in diverting money," which was anticipated to be in the range
of a quarter million pounds.

Florey said his own "impression is that if we press 'Penicillin
Memorial Fund' the Scots might play on that; they would not play on
['Penicillin Research Memorial Fund']. I don't mind putting in brack-
ets underneath 'In memory of the late Dr. Alexander Fleming.' "

Margaret Jennings, however, was strongly opposed to Fleming's
name being in the title. Florey was more sanguine. "If we can keep
the committee in being I think that Mary's will be under control."

It seems likely that it was Margaret who summarized the general
feeling in Oxford, in comments typed on the back of Dunn School
stationery (its use no longer embargoed for anything but the most
important business). She typed Florey's letters and papers and would
have had the stationery at hand.

> I don't think any of the penicillin team here object to anonymity
> although it is only human that they should be pleased when anyone
> shows recognition of their services. . . .
>
> Now no one minds this while everyone remains anonymous but a
> great deal of resentment is likely to be aroused if the names of some
> people were publicly recognized and others left out. . . .
>
> The Duke of Edinburgh is a young and intelligent man. If he has
> made a mistake in sponsoring this national memorial to Fleming then
> now, while he is still young, is the right time for him to learn by his
> mistakes. . . . By all means let him encourage the erection of the statue
> to Fleming. It will in future generations, I imagine, simply be regarded
> as a memorial to the persistent blindness of the British people to those
> who are their benefactors. . . .

Though Florey received far less public acclaim than Fleming, Mellanby had correctly predicted that his contribution would not be unap-
preciated by his colleagues. He was awarded honorary doctorates
from more than a dozen universities and honorary memberships of
many prestigious scientific academies. On the occasion that Fleming
and Florey were honored by the Royal Society of Medicine (not to be
confused with the Royal Society), Fleming biographer L. J. Ludovici

wrote, "Each of them received an ovation the like of which had not before been heard from the usually restrained members sitting in august assembly."

Younger scientists did not offer Florey the same recognition. Maxwell Cowan studied at the Dunn School in the mid-1950s, and he later recalled with considerable amusement the occasion a fellow student with whom he was walking asked, "Who is that codger ahead of us? At breakfast a couple of days ago I saw this chap sitting on his own and he let me join him. I asked him what he was doing. He said he was working on mucus. My God, how sad. Here's a man probably in his sixties, probably at the end of his career, studying mucus." Henry Harris recalls a day in the 1970s that he asked a lecture hall full of Dunn School students if they knew who Howard Florey was. Only six out of about one hundred did.

In the years after Florey and his children returned to England in 1945, Charles was enrolled at Rugby, but Paquita found a place at the Oxford High School for Girls, and so lived at home. This gave her special time with her parents. Ethel "would rest in the afternoon. I'd come home about four o'clock with German homework. I'd make tea and bring it up with four slices of bread or so and she'd take me through the verbs or decline the nouns. She didn't speak German but could look at it. It was a very nice, pleasant, relaxed time."

Paquita had equally pleasant times with her father. Her school was a three-minute walk from home, and so she returned every day for lunch, as did Howard. Usually, she says, he "was not very relaxed . . . because he was often infuriated through the battles that he was fighting over various developments that might be taking place, either in Oxford or further afield. He would come and tell us stories and he was a great storyteller. . . . Day after day. I can remember hilarious lunches. It was great fun because you went back to school laughing away because, maddened though he might be by whatever was happening, he could tell it so well that we all ended up laughing. He was always known for being witty. He also kept a joke book so that when he spoke in public in a formal sense, he prepared himself using [it]."

There were, as well, some pleasant family holidays in Cornwall.

"Dad had a didactic pleasure in teaching. The thing I could excel at was spelling. We would walk around the headlands and he would test me. 'Rhododendron' was one of the words."

In 1960, Florey followed in the footsteps of his mentor Charles Sherrington when he was elected for a five-year term as president of the Royal Society, then the highest honor that could be given a British scientist. Florey mellowed in his later years, and he was a dynamic and innovative president. He was particularly concerned that all the good medical progress was threatened by the massive growth in population brought about in part by so many saved lives.

"I suppose we're all glad now that [penicillin] works," he said in 1967, "but then you've got to see the reverse side of the medal, because I'm now accused of being partly responsible for the population explosion, which is one of the most devastating things that the world has got to face for the rest of the century [although] the tropical medicine people have done much better. People with malaria and people who have controlled intestinal diseases and so on, they're the ones that are responsible for the very big increases in population. . . . So there's a dark side to all medical advance."

In 1963, Florey was made provost (president) of Queen's College, one of the most beautiful of the Oxford University colleges. Ethel lived in the house they built in the nearby village of Old Marston, but Howard often stayed in his comfortable provost's lodgings that, as he described, "look out on a splendid garden with the facade of one of the best and most beautiful libraries in Oxford." He would pore over catalogues to choose which flowers to put around the garden's border; he had a particular fondness for roses and dahlias, and always chose bright colors. When Paquita and her young son Daniel would come for a visit, Paquita recalls that Florey tested him as he had her, to the pleasure of all three. "Daniel has wonderful memories of going around Queens with Grandpa, his hands behind his back, his feet splayed. He had a great interest in forming Daniel. He walked around every day with him, quizzing him on statues, looking at minute changes in flowers."

In 1965, Florey was made a life peer and became Baron Florey of Adelaide and Marston. He also was appointed a member of the Order of Merit, one of the greatest British honors.

Ethel died in September 1966. Howard's angina worsened. He had long hid it from his colleagues for fear that knowledge of it would dilute his authority with pity, but he shared his condition with Margaret. Despite more than twenty-five years of intimacy, a letter he wrote her in November 1966 displays his inherent formality and remove.

Dear Mrs. Jennings,

I have made the will to which this is attached on the supposition that I shall die quite soon. The will places a heavy burden on you and I want to make it clear what I have in mind.

I want you to have first choice among *all* my goods and chattels which are now in the lodgings. As you will probably live in a small house, clearly, you cannot accommodate them all. The things you don't want can be distributed in consultation with Paq and maybe Bertie [who was then working in the United States].

I am sorry you will have so much to do.

Yours ever,
Howard Florey

They were married on June 6, 1967, in the Oxford Registry Office. The only witnesses were James Kent and Margaret's housekeeper. A quiet celebration in Florey's rooms at Queen's College followed, with a few people from the Dunn School along with Heatley and others from the penicillin team. After a short trip to the Caribbean and to New Haven to visit Lucia Fulton, they settled in Oxford, content in each other's company. In Margaret's letter about their relationship she wrote:

Our delight in each other, now that we could always be together, was unbounded. I learned to relax, after the great strains of the preceding years, and felt, and looked, a different woman. There was always time for him, and for us to be together, whatever else might be neglected.

Among Florey's many accomplishments as president of the Royal Society was to raise the money to move it from its longtime home in Burlington House in Piccadilly, where it shared tenancy with, among others, the Royal Academy of Arts. The larger quarters are part of Carleton House Terrace, the row of spectacular Georgian houses designed by the great John Nash, beside the Duke of York steps that lead to Pall Mall. It was formally opened in November 1967. Florey, ailing, was still a lively presence.

Even as his health declined, Florey continued to work until the evening of February 21, 1968, when, at age sixty-nine, he died from a heart attack. A plaque in his honor is embedded in the wall by the door entering the Anglican church in Old Marston, across the street from the house he and Ethel built. The vestry refused to install it inside because Florey was so outspoken in his disbelief. Westminster Abbey was not so adamant. In 1982, a commemorative plaque was put in the floor of the nave, near the one for Charles Darwin and in the company of those for other illustrious scientists.

There was never a party or dinner to celebrate the Oxford team's accomplishment. Instead, they worked on. Norman Heatley continued at the Dunn School until his retirement in 1976. In the 1950s, he worked with Edward Abraham on cephalosporin, until, after six months, Florey inexplicably assigned him to other work in the lab. Once Abraham was granted the patent on the drug, in acknowledgment of Heatley's contribution, he offered him a share in what to date has been royalties in excess of £80 million. Heatley turned this down on the grounds that his modest academic salary met his family's needs. At times in later years he lamented that no other work he did matched the result of penicillin, but how often in a lifetime can one hope to change the world? Until his death at the age of ninety-two on January 5, 2004, he and Mercy lived in Old Marston in the house they shared for over fifty years. In the large back garden are the Lane's Prince Albert apple tree that provided him with a piece of fruit for lunch all those years, and a red Gypsy wagon in which their grandchildren play. In 1978, he was appointed to the Order of the British Empire.

Before Florey left England in 1945 to receive his Nobel in Stockholm, he talked with Edward Abraham about sharing his prize money of a little under £3,000 with the key people who had contributed to the work on penicillin. Abraham advised him not to; if divided a half-dozen ways, it would not amount to much. Instead, Florey brought back sets of blue wineglasses for Heatley, Abraham, and others of the team. Heatley never used his.

"He said he likes to see the color of the wine," Mercy Heatley recalled in 2002. "When some years later a few fell out of the cupboard, he seemed not to mind at all. This is the most I've seen him protest over being ignored."

The Nobel Committee does not divide a prize among more than three people, and in all the discussions over the award for penicillin, Heatley's name seems never to have been mentioned.

"The committee recommends to the faculty, which is made up mainly of clinicians," Henry Harris points out. Heatley's work would likely be more appreciated today, in a time when the Nobel Committee places greater value on direct contribution. "Norman was overlooked in other respects," Harris adds. "He was put up for the Royal Society but the rumor was that people regarded him as just a pair of hands for Florey because of his diffidence. It was a great injustice."

The injustice was considerably ameliorated in 1990, on the occasion of the fiftieth anniversary of penicillin's development into a drug. In honor of his work so long overlooked, Oxford University conferred on Heatley the first honorary Doctor of Medicine degree given in its eight-hundred-year history. The lab in which he worked at the Dunn School is now the Heatley Lab, and Lincoln College has an annual Heatley Lecture, given by a distinguished scientist.

The development of antibiotics is one of the most successful stories in the history of medicine, but it is unclear whether its ending will be a completely happy one. Fleming prophetically warned in his 1945 Nobel lecture that the improper use of penicillin would lead to its becoming ineffective. The danger was not in taking too much; it was in taking too little to kill the bacteria but "enough to educate them to resist penicillin." Penicillin and the antibiotics that followed were prescribed freely for decades not only to treat ailments they could cure but also to fight many others, such as viral infections, that they have no power against. The result of this misuse is strains of bacteria that are now unfazed by them.

This is unfortunate because there are not many ways to fight microbes, and fewer and fewer antibiotics are being developed. In 2002, no new antibacterial drugs came on the market. In 2003, there were two. The reason is largely economic. The Oxford team developed penicillin for a few thousand dollars. It takes as much as $900 million to bring a drug to market today. As antibiotics often are good for only two or three years before bacteria become resistant to them, pharmaceutical companies do not have the financial incentive to develop new ones. When a company loses interest, its researchers adept at developing and testing antibiotics must move to more profitable areas.

The drugs most coveted by pharmaceutical companies are not antibiotics, which people take for ten days every year or two, but rather those taken every day for life, such as the ones for lowering cholesterol or keeping blood pressure in check. The deciphering of the human genome will eventually lead to a new class of drugs tailored for specific uses, but, says Dr. John G. Bartlett, chief of the Division of Infectious Diseases at Johns Hopkins University School of Medicine and one of the foremost experts on antibiotics, "genome drugs are a long way away practically." In the meantime, there is no need for people "to give up on antibiotics. It is still a minority of cases in which they don't work. The notion that bacteria have won or will win is wrong. There will be occasional exceptions to that, and the work with infectious diseases will get more difficult, but we're a long way from antibiotics being useless." Still, he adds, "ten years ago there wasn't a bug we couldn't treat. Resistance does not go backward."

Unlike drugs for AIDS or hepatitis C, such pinpoint treatments were never developed for the fight against bacteria. Antibiotics often are effective against a broad range of microbes, and although many have lost their effectiveness, there are exceptions: Group A *Streptococcus* is as sensitive to penicillin today as it was sixty years ago.

Despite alarming instances of bacterial resistance, antibiotics usually work, fortified by a pipeline of new drugs, which, Bartlett says, "has kept us a few steps ahead." However, he warns that "the dramatic decrease in the production of new drugs coupled with antibiotic abuse" may lead to some bacteria getting a few steps ahead of humans. Even if that happens, he is optimistic that the intellectual means are available to solve the problem, and recent experience backs him. "If there really were a crisis, there would be a way to mobilize the talent to overcome it, like with SARS."

Researchers working to meet that challenge might do well if they recall the efforts of a group of Oxford scientists whose ingenuity was inversely proportional to their financial backing, and who were forced by war to carry their work in their clothes.

NOTES

A NOTE ON THE NOTES

Most of Howard Florey's papers are in the Florey Archives at the Royal Society in London. The catalogue designation is 98 HF. Following the designation are three other numbers. They describe the box, file, and item number of a citation's location. All references to this collection are preceded RS.

Most of Ernst Chain's papers are at the Wellcome Library for the History and Understanding of Medicine, the Wellcome Trust, London. All references to this collection are preceded Wellcome.

The Rockefeller Foundation Archives is housed in the Rockefeller Archive Center, Sleepy Hollow, New York. It is abbreviated RAC. Papers are sorted by record group, series, box, and folder. Thus a citation might be: 1.1, 401, 36, 457.

Edward Abraham's papers were sent in 2003 from the National Catalogue Unit for Archives of Contemporary Scientists (NCUACS), University of Bath, England, to the Bodleian Library, Oxford University. The designation of his collection is NCUACS 103/2/02, and individual items are numbered by folder, for example, D. 168.

Gwyn Macfarlane wrote excellent biographies of both Alexander Fleming and Howard Florey. Reference to *Alexander Fleming: The Man and the Myth*, Cambridge: Harvard University Press, 1984, is Macfarlane (*AF*); reference to *Howard Florey: The Making of a Great Scientist*, Oxford: Oxford University Press, 1979, is Macfarlane (*HF*). Letters to him are cited R. G. Macfarlane.

John Farquhar Fulton's papers are housed at the Yale University Library: Manuscripts and Archives, Sterling Memorial Library and the Historical Library, Cushing/Whitney Medical Library. All correspondence with a folder number, such as 775, are kept in Manuscripts and Archives. All diary citations with a volume number, such as XVII, are kept in the Cushing/Whitney Medical Library.

Material from the Nobel Archives was kindly provided by the Nobel Committee for Physiology or Medicine.

Norman G. Heatley graciously loaned me his personal diaries and citations from them are abbreviated NGH/D. He is abbreviated NGH.

The National Library of Australia is abbreviated NLA.

Howard Walter Florey is abbreviated HWF.

Interviews I conducted are abbreviated EL.

INTRODUCTION: THE RECLAIMED LIFE

1 Details of Anne Miller: Obituary, *The New York Times*, June 9, 1999.

3 *Just what caused infection*: Peter Baldry, *The Battle Against Bacteria: A Fresh Look* (Cambridge: Cambridge University Press, 1976), pp. 1–7.

4 Edward Jenner is considered the father of immunology, and his determination in the face of disbelief in inoculation and open hostility to it brought about a revolution in medicine. But long before his introduction of the cowpox vaccine, inoculation by insertion of smallpox pus into cuts made on the arms and legs was common in the Ottoman Empire and in Africa. In the early 1700s, Cotton Mather and Benjamin Franklin were public advocates of inoculation, and Lady Mary Worley Montagu in Georgian London and Zabdiel Boylston in colonial Boston were catalysts in the inoculation movement.

1: THE QUIET SCOT

7–9 Details of Fleming's early life: Gwyn Macfarlane, *Alexander Fleming: The Man and the Myth* (Cambridge: Harvard University Press, 1984), pp. 9–19.

8 *"He was not . . ."*: E. T. Williams, and Helen M. Palmer, ed., *The Dictionary of National Biography, 1951–60* (London: Oxford University Press, 1971), p. 363.
America Line: Macfarlane (*AF*), p. 21.
family competitions: Macfarlane (*AF*), p. 21; Robert Scott Root-Bernstein, *Discovering* (Cambridge: Harvard University Press, 1989), p. 145.

9 *sum of £250*: Macfarlane (*AF*), pp. 24–25.
seventeen subjects: Ibid. p. 38.
£145 prize: Ibid., pp. 39–46; André Maurois, *The Life of Sir Alexander Fleming, Discoverer of Penicillin*, trans. Gerard Hopkins (New York: E. P. Dutton and Company, 1959), p. 33.

10 *Inoculation Department*: Macfarlane (*AF*), p. 66.

11 Quinine, a white powder from the bark of Andean cinchona trees, kills the parasite that causes malaria. Introduced to Europe by Jesuits around 1640, it is considered the first true chemotherapeutic treatment; the active ingredient was not isolated until 1820.
Syringes of the day: Michael Dunnill, *The Plato of Praed Street: The Life and Times of Almroth Wright* (London: The Royal Society of Medicine Press, 2002), p. 111.
"I play with microbes . . .": Macfarlane (*AF*), p. 246.

12 *underpinning of play*: Root-Bernstein, *Discovering*, p. 147.
    A human body is host: James Gorman, "Aliens Inside Us: A (Mostly Friendly) Bacterial Nation," *New York Times*, April 1, 2003.

13 *casino at Boulogne*: Dunnill, *Plato of Praed Street*, p. 169.

14 *Sir William Watson Cheyne*: Ibid., p. 168.
    The fighting in South Africa: Ibid., 168–69.

15 *"We have, in this war . . ."*: Leonard Colebrook, *Almroth Wright, Provocative Doctor and Thinker* (London: William Heinemann, 1954), p. 72.
    lab at Boulogne: Macfarlane (*AF*), p. 85.
    "I have known . . .": Maurois, *Life of Fleming*, pp. 232–33.
    Fleming examined wound swabs: Macfarlane (*AF*), p. 85.

16–17 *The conventional story*: Macfarlane (*AF*), pp. 118–19.

19 *"the window was seldom . . ."*: Ronald Hare, *The Birth of Penicillin* (London: George Allen and Unwin, 1970), p. 81.
    Repeated attempts: Ibid., p. 78.

20 *Fleming's later paper*: Ibid., p. 66.
    "This is interesting.": Macfarlane (*AF*), p. 99.
    found this dissolving agent: L. J. Ludovici, *Fleming, Discoverer of Penicillin* (London: Andrew Dakers, 1952), pp. 100–1.
    Beyond his own searches: Macfarlane (*AF*), p. 108.

21 *destroyed about 75 percent*: Ibid. (*AF*), p. 107.
    His lectures . . .: Stanley Peart, interview with Dr. Max Blythe, Oxford Brookes University, The Royal College of Physicians and Oxford Brookes University Medical Sciences Video Archive.

22 *Medical Research Club*: Macfarlane, (*AF*), p. 102.
    Root-Bernstein's view: Root-Bernstein, *Discovering*, p. 177.

23 *"Pryce had often . . ."*: Maurois, *Life of Fleming*, p. 125.
    "Therefore mould culture . . .": Macfarlane, (*AF*), p. 121.
    "Now I ask you . . .": Root-Bernstein, *Discovering*, pp. 177–78.

24 *moldy old shoes*: Macfarlane (*AF*), p. 123.

24–25 Molds as folk medicine: H. W. Florey, E. Chain, N. G. Heatley, M. A. Jennings, A. G. Sanders, E. P. Abraham, and M. E. Florey, *Antibiotics* (London: Oxford University Press, 1949), vol. 1, pp. 1–3.

24 *Hippocrates . . . eunuch's fat*: Berton Roueché, "Something Extraordinary," *The New Yorker*, July 28, 1951, p. 28.

25 *"In the inferior . . ."*: Ronald W. Clark, *The Life of Ernst Chain: Penicillin and Beyond* (New York: St. Martin's Press, 1985), p. 26.
    Gratia's work: Lennard Bickel, *Rise Up to Life: A Biography of Howard Walter Florey Who Gave Penicillin to the World* (London: Angus and Robertson, 1972), p. 60.

26 *"The only usable antiseptic . . ."*: Maurois, *Life of Fleming*, p. 131.

26–27 Fleming's tests: Macfarlane (*AF*), p. 128.

27   "*not because of any dislike . . .*": Hare, *Birth of Penicillin*, p. 138.

27–28   Trial on patient: Maurois, *Life of Fleming*, p. 133.

28   Naming penicillin: Ibid., p. 134; Macfarlane (*AF*), p. 123.
Craddock and Ridley's workspace: Hare, *Birth of Penicillin*, p. 55.
"*Ridley had sound . . .*": Maurois, *Life of Fleming*, p. 135.

29   *goal was to make . . . crystals*: Ibid., p. 135.
"*full of hope . . .*": Ibid., pp. 135–36.
"*a bacteriologist . . .*": Ibid., p. 136.
"*He was very shy . . .*": Ibid., pp. 136–37.

30   "*that frightful moment*": Ibid., p. 137.
custom of the Inoculation Department: Ibid., p. 138.
"*not the recording . . .*": Hare, *Birth of Penicillin*, p. 61.

2: THE ROUGH COLONIAL GENIUS

32   "*I endeavoured . . .*": letter, February 22, 1922, HWF to Ethel Hayter Reed, RS 98, HF 287.1.17.

32–33   Florey's early life: Gwyn Macfarlane, *Howard Florey: The Making of a Great Scientist* (Oxford: Oxford University Press, 1979), pp. 30–34.

33   "*Floss*": Charles Florey, interview with EL.
Nature of Australian students: Macfarlane (*HF*), pp. 39–40.
"*Oh, you'd like . . .*" and "*. . . a reasonable thing to do*": HWF, National Library of Australia, Oral History Section, tape 220, April 5, 1967.
Joseph Florey's financial problems: Macfarlane (*HF*), p. 38.
Howard Florey's prize and size of medical school: Ibid., p. 43.

34   "*The teaching of physiology . . .*": HWF, NLA tape.
"*It is far better . . .*": Trevor I. Williams, *Robert Robinson: Chemist Extraordinary* (Oxford: Oxford University Press, 1990), p. 32.
Florey's tennis playing: Bickel, *Rise Up to Life*, pp. 9–10.
Joseph Florey's death and financial crisis: Macfarlane (*HF*), pp. 48–49.
"*there were no opportunities . . .*": HWF, NLA tape.

35   "Women in Medicine" and Ethel Reed: Macfarlane (*HF*), pp. 50–51.
"*You're the only person . . .*": letter, December 21, 1926, HWF to Ethel Reed, RS, 98 HF 287.1.11.
become a student at Magdalen: Macfarlane (*HF*), p. 61.

36   "*one could get away . . .*": HWF, NLA tape.
"*first-rate man . . .*": E. P. Abraham, *Howard Walter Florey: Biographical Memoirs of Fellows of the Royal Society*, 1971, vol. 17, pp. 255–302.
First Class honor: letter, July 7, 1923, HWF to Ethel Reed, RS, 98 HF 287.2.8.
"*Webb*" *in return*: Bickel, *Rise Up to Life*, p. 25.
"*I can see myself . . .*": letter, December 26, 1923, HWF to Ethel Reed, RS, 98 HF 287.2.13.
"*Happiness comes from within . . .*": letter, May 19, 1923, HWF to Ethel Reed, RS, 98 HF 287.2.5.

37 *"I think he just . . ."*: Bickel, *Rise Up to Life*, pp. 25–26.
"perhaps the only man . . .": Henry Harris, *The Balance of Improbabilities* (Oxford: Oxford University Press, 1987), p. 76.
Sherrington's suggestions: Abraham, *Florey.*
"for the excellent . . .": letter, July 12, 1923, Charles Sherrington to HWF, RS, 98 HF 290.2.1.

38 *"There have been such . . ."*: letter, November 7, 1926, Charles Sherrington to HWF, RS, 98 HW 290.2.7.
advice on revisions: letter, April 6, 1929, Charles Sherrington to HWF, RS, 98 HF 290.2.18.
"The thing that tickles . . .": letter, May 25, 1924, HWF to Ethel Reed, RS, 98, HF 287.3.8.
"Gonville is never . . .": letter, September 28, 1924, HWF to Ethel Reed, RS, 98, HF 287.3.23.
"deeply respected . . .": Macfarlane (*HF*), p. 83.

39 *"What I'm most proud of . . ."*: letter, November 13, 1925, HWF to Ethel Reed, RS, 98 HF 287.5.19.

39–40 *"His lifelong interest . . . own cardiac pain"*: Harris, *Balance of Improbabilities*, pp. 98–99.

40 *"Florey was not . . ."*: Bickel, *Rise Up to Life*, p. 24.

42 Howard and Ethel's reunion: Macfarlane (*HF*) pp. 148–50.
Florey's return to Cambridge: Ibid., pp. 151–58.

43 *"became a barrier . . ."*: Ibid., pp. 157–58.
Naming Paquita: Bickel, *Rise Up to Life*, p. 40; Macfarlane (*HF*), pp. 167–68.
most communication was through notes: Macfarlane (*HF*), p. 224.
"Mrs. H. W. Florey . . .": memorandum, 1934, HWF to Ethel Florey, RS, 98 HF 288.3.1.

47 *"There is no pathologist . . ."* and Sheffield professorship: Macfarlane (*HF*), pp. 208–9.
Work of Raistrick, Clutterbuck, and Lovell: Ibid., p. 193.

48 *published their results*: British Medical Journal, 1932, vol. 26, p. 1907.
"a pity . . .": letter, February 7, 1946, Alexander Fleming to HWF, RS, 98 HF 35.12.25.
Eye saved by penicillin broth: Florey et al., *Antibiotics*, vol. II, p. 634.
"uniformly disappointing": Bickel, *Rise Up to Life*, p. 45.

49 Perkin, Ehrlich, and dyes: Simon Garfield, *Mauve* (London: Faber and Faber, 2000), p. 159.
Colebrook, Fleming, and Prontosil: Macfarlane (*AF*), pp. 148–49.
Prontosil's effectiveness: Harry F. Dowling, *Fighting Infection: Conquests of the Twentieth Century* (Cambridge: Harvard University Press, 1977, 2000), p. 107.
Prontosil's limitations: Macfarlane (*AF*), pp. 148–49.

50 Florey's years at Sheffield: Bickel, *Rise Up to Life*, p. 42; Macfarlane (*HF*), p. 218.
a dozen published papers: Abraham, *Florey*.
"I have never . . .": Harris, *Balance of Improbabilities*, p. 75.

3: THE MONEY TALKS

51 Details of Dreyer and Dunn School: S. R. Douglas, *Georges Dreyer: Obituary Notices of Fellows of the Royal Society, 1932–1935*, vol. 1, pp. 569–76.

52 Oxford professors as scholars, not administrators: Harris, *Balance of Improbabilities*, p. 57.
Details of professor's office: Ibid., pp. 163–65.
Dreyer's personal history: Douglas, *Dreyer*.
Standards Laboratory: letter, May 29–30, 1976, A. D. Gardner to R. G. Macfarlane, Wellcome, PP/RGM/F.1/5.
Dreyer's imperiousness: Macfarlane (*HF*), pp. 231–33.

53 Leaked results of Dreyer's TB experiments: Macfarlane (*HF*), pp. 228–29.
Inefficiencies at Dunn School and class size: letter, May 29–30, 1976, A. D. Gardner to R. G. Macfarlane, Wellcome, PP/RGM/F.1/5.
"was beginning to show . . .": Abraham, *Florey*.
Details of election of a new Oxford professor: Macfarlane (*HF*), pp. 233–34.

54 *Sherrington also reported*: letter, October 26, 1934, Charles Sherrington to HWF, RS, 98 HF 290.2.25.
"The most important difference . . .": Roy Porter, *The Greatest Benefit to Mankind* (New York: W. W. Norton and Company, 1998), p. 682.

55 *"In his own special . . ."*: letter, December 13, 1934, Charles Sherrington to Oxford electors, RS, 98 HF 291.5.1.
Mellanby's late arrival: Macfarlane (*HF*), p. 236.
"He told them . . .": Sir Henry Harris, interview with EL.

55–56 Details of Cambridge University elections: Sir Aaron Klug, interview with EL.

56 *"Classics were generally . . . "*: A. D. Gardner, *Some Recollections*, unpublished bound typescript, University College Library, Oxford University.

57 *"Florey had a rather . . ."*: Sir Henry Harris, interview with EL.
"He did not much . . .": Gardner, *Some Recollections*, p. 208.
"ally and supporter": letter, May 29–30, 1976, A. D. Gardner to R. G, Macfarlane, Wellcome, PP/RGM/F.1/5.
"an experimental pathologist . . .": Gardner, *Some Recollections*, p. 207.
"Dreyer's rubbish": letter, May 29–30, 1976, A. D. Gardner to R. G. Macfarlane, Wellcome, PP/RGM/F.1/5.

57–58 Florey's budget: Macfarlane (*HF*), p. 243.

4: THE TEMPERAMENTAL CONTINENTAL

59 Details of Chain's early life and *"I was indoctrinated . . ."*: Ronald W. Clark, *The Life of Ernst Chain: Penicillin and Beyond* (New York: St. Martin's Press, 1985), p. 2.
"it was great . . .": Benjamin Chain, interview with EL.

59–61 Details of Chain's early life: Clark, *Life of Chain*, pp. 5–11.

61 Chain's correspondence with Frederick Gowland Hopkins: E. P. Abraham, *Ernest Chain: Obituary Notices of Fellows of the Royal Society*, 1983, vol. 29, p. 44.

62 *"when pleased his face . . ."*: Clark, *Life of Chain*, pp. 6–7.
"He brought . . ." and Chain's mannerisms: Macfarlane (*HF*), p. 256.
"We haven't much money . . .": Clark, *Life of Chain*, p. 13.

63 *vitalism*: Trevor I. Williams, *Science: A History of Discovery in the Twentieth Century* (Oxford: Oxford University Press, 1990), p. 39.
"one of the most . . .": Clark, *Life of Chain*, p. 14.
"rhubarbative personality": Sir Henry Harris, interview with EL.
"temperamental Continental": *Financial Times*, February 1, 1986.

63–64 *"was very proud . . . 'to retire myself' "* and Chain's lack of regard for colleagues: letter, November 17, 1981, Ashley Miles to Edward Abraham, NCUACS 103/2/02, D 138.

64 *"frequent attacks . . . uncertainty of future"*: Clark, *Life of Chain*, p. 15.
"grotty digs": letter, November 17, 1981, Ashley Miles to Edward Abraham, NCUACS 103/2/02, D 138.
"uprooted and disoriented": Clark, *Life of Chain*, p. 16.

65 *"On the way . . ."*: letter, 1935, unknown friend to Ernst Chain, Wellcome, PP/EC/16/12/35.
Chain did original work: Gerald Jonas, *The Circuit Riders: Rockefeller Money and the Rise of Modern Science* (New York: W. W. Norton and Company, 1989), p. 237.
"Pathology will not . . .": HWF, NLA tape.

66 *"He really has become . . ."*: letter, May 28, 1935, Frederick Gowland Hopkins to HWF, RS, 98, HF 291.8.15.
"You have Soxhlets? . . .": letter, 1975, James Kent to R. G. Macfarlane, Wellcome, PP/RGM; Macfarlane (*HF*), p. 256.
"For the first time . . .": *Nature* 281 (October 25, 1979), pp. 715–17; Jonas, *Circuit Riders*, p. 237.
HWF and Chain's walks: Macfarlane (*HF*), p. 259.

67 *"Periodic fear attacks . . ."*: Clark, *Life of Chain*, p. 20.
"a nervous breakdown . . .": letter, November 17, 1981, Ashley Miles to Edward Abraham, NCUACS 103/2/02, D 138.
Diagnosis of appendicitis and souvenir: Clark, *Life of Chain*, p. 21.

68 *"didn't like to talk . . ."*: Benjamin Chain, interview with EL.

5: THE MICRO MASTER

69   Thomas Heatley's skills: NGH, interview with EL.

69–70   *"being an invalid . . . proud and delighted"*: NGH, interview with Dr. Max Blythe, the Royal College of Physicians and Oxford Brookes University Medical Sciences Video Archive MSVA 192.

70   *"his experimental neatness . . ."*: letter, January 3, 1979, Ernst Chain to R. G. Macfarlane, Wellcome, PP/RGM/F.1/5.

71   *"He had read . . ."*: NGH, interview with Blythe.
Hiring Margaret Jennings: Macfarlane (*HF*), pp. 270–71.

72   *"whose prose style . . ."*: Sir Henry Harris, "The Florey Centenary Lecture: Howard Florey and the Development of Penicillin," September 29, 1998.
Joint papers by HWF and Margaret Jennings: Norman G. Heatley, *The Independent*, November 24, 1994.
Nuffield donation: Jonas, *Circuit Riders*, p. 238.
Rockefeller Foundation endowment: Ibid., p. 80.
"to promote . . ." and Rockefeller Foundation details: Ibid., p. 79.

73   *"philanthropoids . . ."*: Ibid., pp. 63–64.
"a German refugee . . .": letter, May 9, 1936, HWF to Daniel P. O'Brien, RAC, RF 1.1, 401, 36, 457.
"was unable to persuade . . .": Harry Miller Jr., oral history, p. 23, RAC, RF RG 13 vol. XXIII.

74   O'Brien passed on correspondence: Jonas, *Circuit Riders*, p. 240.
"should be carefully . . .": letter, May 27, 1936, W. E. Tisdale to D. P. O'Brien, RF 1.1, 401D, 36, 457.
"the progressive wing . . .": Jonas, *Circuit Riders*, p. 242.
"balances, micro balances . . .": W. E. Tisdale, diaries 1936–37, RAC, RF 12–1.
HWF grant: Grant-in-aid No. 36158, June 26, 1939, RAC, RF 1.1, 401D, 36, 457.

75   Dunn School's uncommon approach: Jonas, *Circuit Riders*, p. 236.
"could hardly believe . . .": Norman Heatley, *Relations with E. Chain*, 1978, Wellcome, GC/48/B2.

75–76   *"trivial example . . . to be useful"*: Ibid.

76   *"with reluctance . . . hang on it"*: Ibid. (The paper referred to is N. G. Heatley, I. Berenblum, and E. Chain, "A New Type of Micro Respirometer," *Biochemistry Journal*, 33, 53, 1939.)
"Some frictions arose . . .": letter, January 3, 1979, Ernst Chain to R. G. Macfarlane, Wellcome, PP/RGM/F.1/5.
"forfeited [his] respect": Heatley, *Relations with E. Chain*.
"the very walls . . .": Bickel, *Rise Up to Life*, p. 49.

77   Chain and Heatley's work and frustration over financial support: Macfarlane (*HF*), p. 285.

Use of Dunn School letterhead paper: letter, n.d., Norman Heatley to R. G. Macfarlane, Wellcome, PP/RGM/F.1/4.

Leslie A. Epstein soon changed his surname to Falk.

"brilliant solution": Macfarlane (*HF*), p. 279.

"chapter of biomedical . . .": Ernst Chain, *Journal of the Royal College of Physicians* 6, 103 (1972); Macfarlane (*HF*), p. 279.

78 *"It is difficult . . ."*: Abraham, *Florey*.

Florey's interest in bacterial antagonism: Macfarlane (*HF*), p. 280.

"No one considers . . .": Florey et al., *Antibiotics*, vol. 1, p. 14.

79–80 *"about 200 references . . . undue difficulties"*: Chain, *Journal of the Royal College of Physicians*; Macfarlane (*HF*), p. 281; Clark, *Life of Chain*, p. 34.

81 *"is subject to . . ."*: David Masters, *Miracle Drug* (London: Eyre and Spottiswoode, 1946), p. 74.

"Remember, no one is alive . . .": letter, January 1, 1978, Ernst Chain to R. G. Macfarlane, Wellcome, PP/RGM/F.1/5.

"Professor Florey . . .": Masters, *Miracle Drug*, pp. 72–74.

Bacillus pyocyaneus: *B. pyocyaneus* had been investigated by several people beginning in 1899. Pyocyaneus, the dried raw material, had been used in clinical trials and was available commercially for animals, but it would prove toxic to human tissue. Trevor I. Williams, *Howard Florey: Penicillin and After* (London: Oxford University Press, 1984), p. 79.

82 *"produced nothing . . . be finished"*: Bickel, *Rise Up to Life*, p. 66.

"found by shaking . . .": Jonas, *Circuit Riders*, p. 276.

"that he was having . . .": Macfarlane (*HF*), p. 289.

83 *"the utmost difficulty . . ."*: Bickel, *Rise Up to Life*, p. 55.

"Oxford medical politics . . . prove himself": Daniel O'Brien diary, May 6, 1937, RAC, RF 12.1.

"was having a very difficult time . . .": W. E. Tisdale diary, June 22, 1936, RAC, RF 12.1.

Funding of MRC and transfer of £10,000: Jonas, *Circuit Riders*, p. 247.

"had undoubtedly . . ." and *"keep this team"*: W. E. Tisdale diary, August 7–20, 1938, RAC, RF 12.1.

Money for scientists faced with tyranny: Jonas, *Circuit Riders*, p. 253.

84 *"The lysozyme question . . ."*: remarks, HWF, August 7, 1944, Yale, JFF 770/30.

"an almost impossible . . .": Bickel, *Rise Up to Life*, p. 61.

6. "WITHOUT HEATLEY, NO PENICILLIN"

85 *"several people in the lab . . ."*: NGH/D, September 27, 1940.

"Air-Raid Precautions . . . scoop and hoe": www.fortunecity.co.uk/meltingpot/oxford/330/cards/cman/html.

86 Hospital preparations in Oxford: Macfarlane (*HF*), p. 291.

"work on lytic substances . . .": letter, January 27 1939, HWF to Edward Mellanby, RS, 98 HF 36.6.1.

Chain head of transfusion service: Bickel, *Rise Up to Life*, p. 70.

Chain forbidden to work on patients: Clark, *Life of Chain*, p. 39.

Work arrangements in Oxford: Macfarlane (*HF*), pp. 291–92.

"*She was very much . . .*": Ibid.

87 HWF's research during 1939: Abraham, *Florey*; Macfarlane (*HF*), p. 294.

Chain's problems with growing penicillin: Macfarlane (*HF*), p. 295.

HWF's wish that he had applied a new name: Williams, *Howard Florey*, p. 96.

88 "*You told me the other day . . .*": letter, circa June 1939, HWF to Edward Mellanby; Bickel, *Rise Up to Life*, p. 71; Macfarlane (*HF*), pp. 296–97.

"*your attempts to get . . .*": letter, June 15, 1939, Edward Mellanby to HWF, RS, 98 HF 36.6.2.

89 Charles Florey's supervising labor: Bickel, *Rise Up to Life*, p. 69.

"*Without Fleming . . .*": Harris, "Florey Centenary Lecture."

Heatley's prior knowledge of Fleming's paper: NGH, interview with Dr. Max Blythe, the Royal College of Physicians and Oxford Brookes University Medical Sciences Video Archive MSVA 192.

"*I understand now . . .*": letter, January 3, 1979, Ernst Chain to R. G. Macfarlane, Wellcome, PP/RGM/F.1/5.

"*It is very unfortunate . . .*": letter, October 6, 1939, HWF to H. M. Miller, RAC, RF 1.1, 401D, 36, 457.

90 "*daily work was much pleasanter . . .*": NGH, Wellcome, GC/48/B2.

"*I enclose some proposals . . .*": letter, September 6, 1939, HWF to Edward Mellanby; Macfarlane (*HF*), pp. 298–300.

91 The antibacterial soil organism referred to in Florey's proposal is gramicidin, which quickly showed it was too toxic for humans.

"*airy optimism*": Macfarlane (*HF*), pp. 298–300.

"*People sometimes think . . .*": HWF, NLA tape.

92 "*sensitive, lonely, unsure of himself . . .*": E. P. Abraham, *Dictionary of National Biography*, Lord Blake and C. S. Nicholls, eds. (Oxford: Oxford University Press, 1981).

"*a glance at his . . .*": Harris, *Balance of Improbabilities*, p. 62.

"*media for growing . . .*": letter, September 6, 1939, HWF to Edward Mellanby; Macfarlane (*HF*), p. 298.

"*You can assume . . .*": letter, September 8, 1939, Edward Mellanby to HWF; Macfarlane (*HF*), p. 300.

"*naturally occurring . . .*" and "those little bits . . .": Clark, *Life of Chain*, p. 40.

93 "*invaded*": NGH, speech to Lord Florey Society, October 28, 1997. Courtesy of Norman Heatley.

"*naturally produced . . .*": Jonas, *Circuit Riders*, p. 267.

"*raised his eyebrows . . .*": HWF, NLA tape.

93–94 "*In spite of the uncertainties . . .*": letter, November 6, 1939, H. M. Miller to Warren Weaver, RAC, RF 1.1, 401D, 36, 457.

94   *"RF officers customarily . . ."*: Jonas, *Circuit Riders*, p. 268.
Miller's cable: Ibid., p. 268.
Rockefeller board and American isolationism: Ibid., p. 271.

94–95   HWF and Chain proposal to Rockefeller: Florey et al., *Antibiotics*, vol. 2, p. 636; RS, 98 HF 36.17.1.

95   RF approval: letter, February 19, 1940, H. M. Miller to HWF, RAC, RF 1.1, 401D, 36, 458.
"magnificent assistance": letter, February 27, 1940, HWF to H. M. Miller, RAC, RF 1.1, 401D, 36, 458.

96   *His "sole abiding . . ."*: Abraham, *Chain*, pp. 43–91.
HWF obtains MRC grant for Abraham: Williams, *Robert Robinson*, p. 123.
Ethel dividing mattress: letter, NGH to R. G. Macfarlane, Wellcome, PP/RGM/F.1/4.
Work on penicillin after NGH took over growing mold: Florey et al., *Antibiotics*, vol. 2, p. 644.

97   *"He was a most versatile . . ."*: Macfarlane (*HF*), pp. 302–3.
"The only practical information . . .": letter, 1974, NGH to R. G. Macfarlane, Wellcome, PP/RGM/F.1/4.

97–98   Assaying a chemical substance and Heatley's methods: NGH, interview with Jeffrey L. Sturchio, October 25, 1989, Rockefeller University. Courtesy NGH.

99   *"The noise . . ."*: Williams, *Howard Florey*, pp. 98–99.

100   *"my beautiful working hypothesis . . ."*: E. B. Chain, "Thirty Years of Penicillin Therapy," *Proceedings of the Royal Society*, B. 179:293–319, 1971.

100–1   Chain and penicillin separation: David Wilson, *In Search of Penicillin* (New York: Alfred A. Knopf, 1976), p. 158.

101   Heatley's broth: Ibid., p. 175; Bickel, *Rise Up to Life*, p. 83.
Fortunate to have a milligram of penicillin: Masters, *Miracle Drug*, p. 78.

102   *"[Our] increasing friction . . ."*: NGH, Wellcome, GC/48/B2.
"I had leaped . . .": NGH/D.

103   *"On arrival . . ."* and *"P is slightly . . ."*: Ibid.
"Had a discussion . . .": Ibid., March 18, 1940.
Florey's style in the lab: Macfarlane (*HF*), p. 305.
"Do the experiment": Ibid., p. 361.
"genuinely disliked theory . . .": Harris, *Balance of Improbabilities*, pp. 75–76.

104   *"laughably simple . . ."* and *"Then if you think . . ."*: N. G. Heatley, "In Memorium, H. W. Florey," *Journal of General Microbiology*, vol. 61, no. 3 (1970), p. 229.
"I must state categorically . . .": letter, January 3, 1979, Ernst Chain to R. G. Macfarlane, Wellcome, PP/RGM/F.1/5.
Florey's wish that the conversation had been taped: NGH, Wellcome, GC/48/B.1.

105 *"This was once again . . ."*: letter, January 3, 1979, Ernst Chain to R. G. Macfarlane, Wellcome, PP/RGM/F.1/5.

106 *"anything that happened . . ."*: Sir Henry Harris, interview with EL.

106–7 Details of extraction: Masters, *Miracle Drug*, p. 95.

107 *"Röentgen's original X-ray tube . . ."*: Williams, *Howard Florey*, p. 120.
"The rubbish dumps aren't . . .": NGH, interview with EL.

107–8 Industry and imagination of innovative scientists: Root-Bernstein, *Discovering*, p. 396.

108–9 Operation of Heatley's apparatus: Masters, *Miracle Drug*, pp. 92–94; Florey et al., *Antibiotics*, vol. 2, p. 644.

109 *"In the opinion . . ."*: Florey et al., *Antibiotics*, vol. 2, p. 644.

110 *"a very nice brown powder . . ."*: Clark, *Life of Chain*, p. 43.
Heatley's witches' feast greeting: Megan Nurser, interview with EL.
"The last time I appeared . . .": letter, January 3, 1979, Ernst Chain to R. G. Macfarlane, Wellcome, PP/RGM/F.1/5.

111 *"Florey sometimes threw off . . ."*: Clark, *Life of Chain*, p. 47.
"We seem to be . . ." and *"Well it seems . . ."*: letter, April 19, 1968, R. L. Vollum to E. P. Abraham, NCUACS 103/2/02, D 84.
"Although he was obviously . . .": Harris, *Balance of Improbabilities*, p. 75.
"Of course, there happened . . .": NGH, interview with EL.

112 *"this was the crucial . . ."*: Clark, *Life of Chain*, p. 48; Bickel, *Rise Up to Life*, p. 67.
"you were too busy . . .": Clark, *Life of Chain*, p. 48.

113 *"He was so skeptical . . ."* and *an enormous antibacterial . . .* : Ibid., p. 49.

7. EIGHT MICE

115 Cellular change: A. D. Gardner, "Morphological Effects of Penicillin on Bacteria," *Nature*, 146 (1940), pp. 837–38.

116 Penicillin's various effectiveness: E. P. Abraham, E. Chain, "An Enzyme from Bacteria Able to Destroy Penicillin," *Nature* 146 (1940), p. 837.
Thirty thousand tuberculosis deaths: Macfarlane (*HF*), p. 311.
Tuberculosis most widespread disease: William H. McNeill, *Plagues and Peoples* (New York: Anchor Books, 1998), p. 288.
Tuberculosis kills two hundred people per hour: *New York Times*, April 30, 2003.

117 Heatley's free time activities: NGH, Wellcome, GC/48/B.1.
"I had to do . . .": Gardner, *Some Recollections*, p. 212.
"I used to call . . .": Ibid., pp. 209–10.

118 *"an indication of the urgency . . ."*: NGH, "In Memorium."

118–19 Details of injections: Florey et al., *Antibiotics*, vol. 2., p. 638.
Heatley's activities: NGH/D, May 25, 1940.

119 *"As the events . . .":* NGH, interview with EL.
"the non-toxicity . . .": Florey et al., *Antibiotics*, vol. 2., p. 638.

120 *"relief, joy, happiness . . .":* NGH, interview with EL.
"It looks . . .": Bickel, *Rise Up to Life*, p. 98.

120–21 *"Lifeboats from liners . . .":* Winston Churchill, *Their Finest Hour* (New York: Houghton Mifflin Company, 1949), p. 101.

121 Chamberlain and Halifax and *"nations which went down . . .":* John Keegan, *Winston Churchill* (New York: Viking, 2002), p. 134.

122 *"As I told you . . .":* letter, June 29, 1940, HWF to Edward Mellanby, RS, 98 HF 35.1.3.
"chemical work . . .": letter, July 16, 1940, Edward Mellanby to HWF, RS, 98 HF 35.1.5.

122–23 Details for Kent's work: Masters, *Miracle Drug*, p. 82.
Details of mouse experiment and *"There could be . . .":* Gardner, *Some Recollections*, p. 211.

126 Fleming's house bombed: Macfarlane (*AF*), p. 189.

127 *"I'm afraid your parents . . .":* letter, March 24, 1966, HWF to Charles Florey, courtesy of Charles Florey.
"Howard had a tenderly . . .": Margaret Florey, memo dated April 4, 1968, and deposited in RS, 98 HF 297.11.1.

128–29 *"This is my surmise . . . with a crocodile":* Harris, interview with EL.

129 *"fight with her . . .":* NGH, interview with EL.
"It puzzled me . . .": letter, November 8, 1976, A. D. Gardner to R. G. Macfarlane, Wellcome, PP/RGM/F.1/5.

130 *"Florey dominated . . . and working late":* Harris, interview with EL.

131 *"tell anybody . . .":* Charles Florey, interview with EL.
"may be the reason . . .": Paquita Florey McMichael, interview with EL.
"Dad didn't like fuss . . .": Macfarlane (*HF*), p. 321.
Emotions upon departure: Paquita Florey McMichael, interview with Max Blythe, Oxford Brookes University, the Royal College of Physicians and Oxford Brookes University Medical Sciences Video Archive.

132 OXFORD SAILING LIST . . . : cable, July 9, 1940, J. F. Fulton to HWF, Yale, JFF 775.
VERY MANY THANKS . . . : cable, HWF to J. F. Fulton, Yale, JFF 775.
Fulton's biographical information: obituary, *New York Times*, May 30, 1960. Apart from his position as professor of physiology, Fulton helped to develop Yale Medical School as a center of aeromedical research and during World War II the Yale Aeromedical Research Unit devised a suit for high-altitude flying. Fulton had lifelong interest in rare medical books and in the

history of medicine, and he was primarily responsible for the development of Yale's Cushing/Whitney Medical Library, which was the recipient of his large personal collection.

"*in-laws are rotten . . .*": letter, January 1, 1926, HWF to Ethel Reed, RS, 98 HF 287.6.1.

Fulton in Montreal: letter, July 24, 1940, J. F. Fulton to HWF, Yale, JFF, 775.

"*Paquita Florey, 10 . . .*": *New Haven Journal and Courier*, July 25, 1940.

133 "*My Dear John and Lucia . . .*": letter, July 21, 1940, HWF to John and Lucia Fulton, Yale, JFF 775.1.

134 "*Paquita is a great . . .*": letter, August 5, 1940, J. F. Fulton to HWF, Yale JFF 775.

134–35 "*a lifestyle that excluded them . . .*": details of Fultons' entertaining and

135 Paquita's feelings: Paquita Florey McMichael, interview, EL.

"*You have never . . .*": letter, May 7, 1956, J. F. Fulton to HWF, RS, 98 HF 197.52.

8: BLITZED

136 "*The months spent . . .*": Florey et al., *Antibiotics*, vol. 2, p. 645.

137 Details of chromatography: *The Lancet*, August 16, 1941.
Reason to produce a salt of penicillin: Wilson, *In Search of Penicillin*, p. 181.

137–38 Increased resistance to penicillin: *The Lancet*, August 16, 1941.

139 "*It has not escaped . . .*": *Nature*, no. 4356, April 25, 1953.
"*Penicillin has not . . .*" and "*Fortunately . . .*": Florey et al., *Antibiotics*, vol. 2, p. 642.

140 "*I forwarded a copy . . .*": letter, August 27, 1940, Edward Mellanby to HWF, RS, 98 HF 36.6.13.

141 "*Thank you for your letter . . .*": letter, August 29, 1940, HWF to Edward Mellanby, RS, 98 HF 36.6.14.

143 "*I think you have given . . .*": letter, September 3, 1940, Edward Mellanby to HWF, RS, 98 HF 36.6.15.
Fleming's publications: Macfarlane (*AF*), p. 147.
Florey's publications: Abraham, *Florey*.

143–44 Work discussed with Fleming: NGH, Wellcome, GC/48/B.1.

144 "*with my old penicillin*": Macfarlane (*HF*), p. 323.
"*It only remains . . .*": letter, November 15, 1940, Alexander Fleming to HWF, RS, 98 HF 35.12.1.

145 "*Soon hundreds of two-liter flasks . . .*": Gladys L. Hobby, *Penicillin: Meeting the Challenge* (New Haven: Yale University Press, 1985), p. 72.
Czapek-Dox medium consists of glucose in water with added salts of sodium, potassium, manganesese, and iron.

"*establish that it would . . .*" and incubation in amphitheater: Hobby, *Penicillin*, p. 75.

'GIANT' GERMICIDE . . . : *New York Times*, May 6, 1941.

GERM KILLER FOUND . . . : *Philadelphia Evening Bulletin*, May 5, 1941.

145–46 Work of Herrell and Waksman: Hobby, *Penicillin*, p. 79.

146 Work by Rake and Pfizer: Ibid., p. 75.

145–47 Work in America on penicillin by Reid and others: W. H. Helfand, H. B. Woodruff, K. M. H. Coleman, and D. L. Cowan, "Wartime Industrial Production of Penicillin in the United States," in *The History of Antibiotics: A Symposium*, ed. John Parascandola (Madison: American Institute of the History of Pharmacy, 1980).

147–48 NGH and new vessels: NGH/D.

148 "*Heatley has gone . . .*": letter, October 31, 1941, HWF to Edward Mellanby, RS, 98 HF 36.4.5.

Five hundred ordered, then another two hundred: NGH, Wellcome, GC/48/B.1 and NGH/D.

148–49 Abraham's pistol: NGH, interview with EL.

149 First vessels driven through snowstorm: Florey et al., *Antibiotics*, vol. 2, p. 643.

"*What a year! . . .*": NGH/D.

149–50 Details of Ruth Callow Parker: interview with EL.

150 Details of Megan Lancaster Nurser: interview with EL.

151 "*The place was full . . .*": Ruth Parsons, interview with EL.

"*We had fun . . .*": Megan Nurser, interview with EL.

"*excitable. He paced . . .*": Ruth Parsons, interview with EL.

152 "*There would have been . . .*": Macfarlane (*HF*), p. 184.

153 "*I am surprised . . .*": Gardner, *Some Recollections*, p. 212.

Administration to Mrs. Akers: Florey et al., vol. 2, p. 647.

January 27: There is disagreement among historians as to whether the date was January 17 or January 27. A chronology compiled by Florey (RS, 98 HF 34.6.6) lists January 27 and that is the date that appears in *Antibiotics II* (p. 647). Wilson and Macfarlane contend January 17 was actually the date because although there is no record in the patient's medical file of when the shot was given; her temperature chart, kept at the foot of the bed, shows a spike on January 17, which they take as evidence of the injection (Wilson, *In Search of Penicillin*, pp. 162–63). But if it was carried out on January 27, it seems equally possible that in the excitement of the test, as no one recorded the administration of the penicillin in the patient's records, they might also have omitted recording her reaction to it. In a 1984 article in the *British Medical Journal*, Fletcher uses January 17, based on Wilson's sleuthing. Absent solid proof one way or the other, I've chosen to stick with Florey's date. Heatley's diary, normally a fount of events and dates, shows nothing for this period because from January 15 to 19 and January 21 to

27 he was in bed with the flu, as were several others in the lab. Florey also was out sick for some days in this time. On January 20, the one day Heatley did come in, there is no mention of a toxicity test having been done. Rather, he recorded only that he "staggered down to the lab at 11 o'clock, and worked up about 30 litres of P in the machine. . . . Chain kept buzzing round and making a nuisance of himself . . . went back to bed before dinner" (NGH/D).

154   *"Every hospital . . ."*: Charles Fletcher, *British Medical Journal* 289, December 22–29, 1984, pp. 1721–23.

     "bandaging and rest . . .": Charles Fletcher, interview with Max Blythe, Oxford Brookes University, the Royal College of Physicians and Oxford Brookes University Medical Sciences Video Archive.

154–56   Albert Alexander: Florey et al., *Antibiotics*, vol. 2, p. 647; HWF, August 7, 1944, Yale, JFF, 776/31.

155   *"Chain dancing with excitement . . ."*: BBC broadcast, December 17, 1968, Abraham, NCUACS 103/2/02, D 101.

156   *"The attempt to treat . . ."*: *The Lancet*, August 16, 1941.

     "typical of those . . .": Florey et al., *Antibiotics*, vol. 2, p. 648.

9: "WILL THESE PLANS COME TO GRIEF?"

157   *"mobilized the English language . . ."*: Keegan, *Winston Churchill*, pp. 142–43.

158   Dale a go-between: Macfarlane (*HF*), p. 334.

159   Weaver recovering from accident: Jonas, *Circuit Riders*, p. 302.

     "This project, if it were indeed . . .": Warren Weaver diaries 1941–1946, RAC, RF RG 12-1, box 68, p. 25.

     "The only way . . .": letter, April 1941, Edward Mellanby to HWF; Macfarlane (*HF*), p. 337; Clark, *Life of Chain*, p. 68.

159–60   Details of arrangements for trip to America: Jonas, *Circuit Riders*, p. 303.

160   *"It seems to me very undesirable . . ."*: letter, April 16, 1941, HWF to Edward Mellanby, RS, 98 HF 35.10.3.

161   *"I am entirely . . ."*: letter, April 25, 1941, Alexander Fleming to HWF, RS, 98 HF 35.10.5.

     "I do not see . . .": letter, April 23, 1941, Edward Mellanby to HWF, RS, 98 HF 35.10.4.

     "is in sufficiently close touch . . .": letter, November 29, 1940, Alexander Fleming papers, British Library, 6113 vol. 8, general correspondence 1930–1944.

     "I think I told . . .": letter, February 21, 1941, Alexander Fleming to J. S. White, Alexander Fleming papers, British Library, 6113 vol. 8, general correspondence 1930–1944.

162   Fleming not particularly involved with Parke, Davis work: Macfarlane (*AF*), p. 181.

163 SARS patent applications: Anthony Regalado, "Scientists' Hunt for SARS Cure Turns to Competition for Patents," *Wall Street Journal*, May 5, 2003.
"*To the electron* . . .": Michael Riordan and Lillian Hoddeston, *Crystal Fire: The Invention of the Transistor and the Birth of the Information Age* (New York: Norton, 1997).

163–64 "*I could not believe* . . ." and "*The people have paid* . . .": Bickel, *Rise Up to Life*, p. 134.

164 "*quite apart from economic* . . ." through ". . . *whole status of my fellow refugees*": E. Chain, "Annotations to the History of Penicillin Discovery," published in Florey et al., *Antibiotics*.
"*There was a strong streak* . . .": W. Maxwell Cowan, interview with EL.

165 "*having got his decision* . . .": John Fulton diary, Yale, JFF.
"*I should be very glad* . . .": letter, May 12 1941, HWF to Edward Mellanby, Abraham, NCUACS 103/2/02, D 67.

166 "*I think you had better* . . .": letter, May 14, 1941, Edward Mellanby to HWF, Abraham, NCUACS 103/2/02, D 67.
"*an ideal case* . . .": NGH/D.

166–68 Treatment of patients: Florey et al., *Antibiotics*, vol. 2, pp. 648–49.

167 Amount of penicillin used: *Science* 253 (August 16, 1991), p. 735.

168 "*it tasted foul*": Bickel, *Rise Up to Life*, p. 132.
"*It was clear* . . . *clinical trial.*": Florey et al., *Antibiotics*, vol. 2, p. 649.

169 "*polish up the bags.*": NGH/D, May 30, 1941.

169–70 "*the penicillin work* . . . *I am concerned*" and "*No other word* . . . *this man forever*": letter, January 3, 1979, Ernst Chain to R. G. Macfarlane, Wellcome, PP/RGM/F.1/5.

170 "*Neither man* . . .": Jonas, *Circuit Riders*, p. 281.
"*unconscious habit of seeing* . . .": Clark, *Life of Chain*, p. 69.
"*I always have considered* . . .": letter, January 10, 1979, Ernst Chain to R. G. Macfarlane, Wellcome, P/RGM/F.1/5.

10: THE FRIEND IN DEED

171 "*The sensation* . . .": letter, June 28, 1941, HWF to Ethel Reed Florey, RS, 98 HF 34.19.8.

172 "*The food I had better not mention* . . ." and details of Lisbon: letter, HWF to Ethel Reed Florey, RS, 98 HF 34.19.8.
Details of Clipper interior, etc.: www.flyingclippers.com.

173 Details of Catherine Dreyfus, cargo on Clipper, and " '*medical business*' . . .": *New York Times*, July 3, 1941.
"*We are always* . . .": Alan Gregg, oral history, p. xii, RAC, RF RG 13 box 2.

174 "*I remember him best of all* . . .": Bickel, *Rise Up to Life*, p. 141.
Details of meeting with Gregg: NGH/D, July 3, 1941, and NGH, RS, 98 HF 46.1.6.

175–77 Details of HWF and NGH at Fultons': J. F. Fulton diary, vol. 17, July 6, 1941, Yale, JFF.

176 The chairman of the National Research Council Committee on Infectious Diseases was Dr. Francis Blake.

177–78 First time to relax, accommodations in Washington, D.C., and details of Thom: NGH/D.

178 THOM HAS INTRODUCED . . . and PAN SETUP AND ORGANISMS . . . : Hobby, Penicillin, p. 89.

179 Additional Rockefeller grant: Jonas, Circuit Riders, p. 304.
I KNOW IT WILL . . . : Hobby, Penicillin, p. 89.
Terms of agreement on patents: September 29, 1941, RS, 98 HF 46.3.36 and 37.

180 "the gutters overrunning . . .": NGH, interview with EL.
"My dear Girl . . .": letter, July 22, 1941, HWF to Ethel Reed Florey, RS, 98 HF 34.19.1.

182–83 Gita Burkhard's achievements: NGH/D, July 19, 1941.

183 "typical town of the Middle West . . .": letter, August 21, 1941, NGH to George Glister, courtesy of Norman Heatley.

184 "a relief . . .": NGH/D.

185 "we were smarter . . .": Bickel, Rise Up to Life, p. 147.
"had lived so much . . .": NGH/D.

186 "a carpet bag salesman . . .": NGH/D.
"Florey is a scientist . . .": Bickel, p. 152.

187 "Without Richards . . .": Sir Henry Harris, interview with EL.
"the pay off . . . from having worked in the States": HWF, NLA tape.

188 "The country might . . .": Hare, Birth of Penicillin, p. 167.
"the problem . . .": Ibid., p. 173.

189 Florey's regard for Defries: Ibid., p. 173; Bickel, Rise Up to Life, p. 150.
Drug companies leery of risk: Hobby, Penicillin, pp. 109–10.

190–91 Details of travel: NGH/D.
"Howard . . . set off this morning . . ." and "Howard . . . returned exhausted": John F. Fulton diary, vol. 17, September 13 and 14, 1941, Yale, JFF.

191 October 8 meeting: A. N. Richards, "Penicillin Production in the United States, 1941–1946," Nature 201, no. 4918 (February 1, 1964): pp. 441–45.

191–92 Details of Woodruff's call and "to work in the lab . . .": letter, October 12, 1941, NGH to HWF, courtesy NGH.

192 "for fear it should reach . . .": letter, October 22, 1941, NGH to HWF, Wellcome, GC/48/D.1.
"as keen as mustard . . .": NGH/D, October 21, 1941.
"more to help . . .": letter, NGH to HWF, Wellcome, GC/48/D.1.

192–93 Details of Peoria: letter, November 21, 1941, NGH to HWF, courtesy NGH.

194 *"I arrived back intact . . ."*: letter, October 1941, HWF to NGH, Wellcome, GC/48/D.2.

"There had been . . .": note on manuscript, 1977, Margaret Florey to R. G. Macfarlane, Wellcome, PP/RGM/F.1/4.

"I cannot recollect . . .": letter, January 3, 1979, Ernst Chain to R. G. Macfarlane, Wellcome, PP/RGM/F.1/5.

195 *"We have lengthened the tube . . ."*: letter, November 17, 1941, HWF to NGH, RS, 98 HF 36.1.14.

"We had a visit from Glaxo . . .": letter, November 21, 1941, HWF to NGH, RS, 98 HF 36.1.15.

196 Details of morgue and *"for a post-mortem . . ."*: Masters, *Miracle Drug*, pp. 122–23.

largest penicillin extraction plant in Britain: Wilson, *In Search of Penicillin*, p. 184; Macfarlane (*HF*), p. 343.

11: THE KILO THAT NEVER CAME

198 *"I shall not . . ."*: letter, January 11, 1942, HWF to NGH, RS, 98 HF 36.1.25.

199 *"You may be interested . . ."*: letter, February 6, 1941, HWF to NGH with postscript by Margaret Jennings, RS, 98 HF 36.1.28.

200 *"a corpse retriever"*: Macfarlane (*HF*), p. 345.

"it is useless . . .": The Lancet, March 27, 1943.

Penicillin shared with Bodenham: Macfarlane (*AF*), p. 196.

201 *"having to do a good deal . . ."*: letter, March 29, 1942, HWF to J. F. Fulton, Yale, JFF 775.31.

"Firstly, thank you for the 5g . . .": letter, April 13, 1942, HWF to NGH, RS, 98 HF 36.1.34.

"This of course we regard . . .": letter, December 15, 1942, HWF to J. H. Burn, RS, 98 HF 35.1.22.

202 *"other firms who have made . . ."*: A. N. Richards, "Penicillin Production in the United States, 1941–1946," *Nature* 201, no. 4918 (February 1, 1964), pp. 441–45.

203 *"could not get into . . ."*: *New Haven Register*, March 11, 1962.

"What would you recommend? . . .": NGH, Sturchio interview.

"the temperature charts . . .": NGH/D, March 22, 1942.

204 Raper's work: Richards, "Penicillin Production"; Wilson, *In Search of Penicillin*, p. 199.

"as something of a betrayal . . .": NGH, interview with EL.

206 *"He is going . . ."*: letter, March 12, 1942, HWF to A. Landsborough Thomson, RS, 98 HF 36.4.32.

"investigating the antibacterial . . .": letter, June 25, 1942, HWF to A. Landsborough Thomson, RS, 98 HF 36.4.60.

"for the chit for the iron . . .": letter, August 17, 1942, HWF to D. K. Chalmers, RS, 98 HF 36.4.69.

"if you could give . . .": letter, March 27, 1943, HWF to A. L. Thomson, RS, 98 HF 36.4.85.

"There is, for me, no doubt . . .": letter, August 2, 1942, HWF to Charles Sherrington, Charles Sherrington Collection, University of British Columbia; Macfarlane (*HF*), p. 346.

207 *Only the development of the atom bomb*: Jonas, *Circuit Riders*, p. 305.
Fleming asks HWF's opinion: Wilson, *In Search of Penicillin*, pp. 214–15; Macfarlane (*AF*), pp. 193–94.

207–8 Details for Lambert: Masters, *Miracle Drug*, pp. 133–34.

208 Rabbit died: Macfarlane (*AF*) p. 194.
"I am rather a pessimist . . .": letter, August 16, 1942, Alexander Fleming to HWF, RS, 98 HF 35.12.3.
"Temperature normal . . .": letter, August 28, 1942, Alexander Fleming, to HWF, RS, 98 HF 35.12.4.

12: THE LAUREL WREATH OF CREDIT

212 *"may give them ten minutes"*: Bickel, *Rise Up to Life*, p. 173.

213 *"I was very glad . . ."*: letter, September 2, 1942, Alexander Fleming to HWF, RS, 98 HF 35.12.6.

214 *"You cannot deplore . . ."*: letter, September 7, 1942, Alexander Fleming to HWF, RS, 98 HF 35.12.7.

215 *"Fleming Myth"*: Macfarlane (*AF*), p. 203.
misinformation and exaggerations: W. Howard Hughes, *Alexander Fleming and Penicillin* (Hove, Sussex: Priory Press, 1974), p. 73.

216 *"The British hospitals . . ."*: Bickel, *Rise Up to Life*, p. 171.
"Florey, well known . . .": Wilson, *In Search of Penicillin*, p. 235.

217 Details of September 25 meeting: Ibid., pp. 222–23.

218 *"Did your officers . . ."*: letter, October 29, 1942, HWF to Director General, BBC, RS, 98 HF 247 1.2.
". . . I have now had . . .": letter, November 9, 1942, Joint Director General, BBC, to HWF, RS, 98 HF 247.1.5.

219 *"It is clear . . ."*: letter, November 13, 1942, HWF to Joint Director General, BBC, RS, 98 HF 247 1.6.
"Dear Sir Henry . . .": letter, December 11, 1942, HWF to Sir Henry Dale, RS, 98 HF 38.3.1.

220 *"My dear Florey . . ."*: letter, December 17, 1942, Sir Henry Dale to HWF, RS, 98 HF 38.3.2.

221 Chain particularly aggrieved: Macfarlane (*AF*), p. 202.

222 War Production Board assistance: Richards, "Penicillin Production."
"One was so successful . . .": Hare, *Birth of Penicillin*, p. 177.

222–23 Exponential production of penicillin in America: Richards, "Penicillin Production."

223 *"Doctor, will all these things . . ."*: Vannevar Bush, "Alfred Newton Richards . . . Some Observations," RS, 98 HF 42.12.44.
Success by Pfizer scientists: Wilson, *In Search of Penicillin*, p. 206.
Solving technical problems: Berton Roueché, "Something Extraordinary," *The New Yorker*, July 28, 1951, p. 32.
Pfizer's success: Wilson, *In Search of Penicillin*, p. 210.
Cost of penicillin: Ibid., p. 203.

224 *"Can penicillin be used. . . ."*: H. W. Florey and H. Cairns, "Special Report," RS, 98 HF 34.11.12; Bickel, *Rise Up to Life*, pp. 199–200.

224–25 Details of Lieutenant Carr: RS, 98 HF 34.16 and 34.11.1, pp. 19–20.

225 *"that it was far . . ."*: Ibid.

226 *"It's murder . . ."*: Wilson, *In Search of Penicillin*, p. 226.
"Give us sulphonamides . . .": Florey and Cairns, "Special Report."
"We are now established . . .": letter, July 25, 1943, HWF to Ethel Reed Florey, RS, 98 HF 34.18.16.

227 *"Results on the whole . . ."*: letter, August 14, 1943, HWF to Ethel Reed Florey, RS, 98 HF 34.18.18.
"Ten cases of resistant . . .": letter, August 8, 1943, HWF to Ethel Reed Florey, RS, 98 HF 34.18.17.
"it was just like turning . . .": Bickel, *Rise Up to Life*, pp. 201–2.

228 *"This valuable drug . . ."*: J. Howie, *British Medical Journal* 2 (1979), p. 1631; Macfarlane (*AF*), p. 197.

13: THE THINKING IN STOCKHOLM

230 *"When I learned that Churchill . . ."*: Bickel, *Rise Up to Life*, p. 211.

231 Sanders's observations of trip: Gordon Sanders, diary, RS, 98 HF 48.2.
"One flies up . . .": letter, April 30, 1944, HWF to J. F. Fulton, RS, 98 HF 776.18.

232 *"Every day the Peruvian . . ."*: letter, HWF to J. F. Fulton, Yale, JFF 776.18.
"I get the greatest . . ." and *"I'm strenuously trying . . ."*: letter, HWF to J. F. Fulton, Yale, JFF 776.18.
"the spectacle of everybody . . .": letter, May 10 1944, HWF to Hilda Florey Gardner, RS, 98 HF 290.1.1.
Time matched donation: Macfarlane (*AF*), p. 205.

233–34 *"the unscrupulous campaign . . . with astonishing properties"*: letter, June 19, 1944, HWF to Edward Mellanby, RS, 98 HF 36.4.107.

234 *"Apart from the chemistry . . ."*: NGH, Sturchio interview.
"Florey was a practical . . .": Sir Henry Harris, interview with EL.
"Immense tracts . . . ": Harris, *Balance of Improbabilities*, p. 85.
"But Florey had . . .": Harris, "Florey Centenary Lecture."

235 *"a difficult position . . ."*: letter, June 20, 1944, Edward Mellanby to HWF, RS, 98 HF 36.4.108.

236 "*I gather that it is proposed . . .*": letter, August 10, 1944, Lord Moran to Anthony de Rothschild, Wellcome, PP/CMW.

"*I feel sure . . .*": letter, August 15, 1944, Anthony de Rothschild to Lord Moran, Wellcome, PP/CMW.

237 "*His Majesty, the King . . .*": Ludovici, *Fleming, Discoverer of Penicillin,* p. 201.

daily afternoon tea: Macfarlane (*AF*), p. 209.

Wright's behavior: Hughes, *Alexander Fleming,* pp. 82–83; Macfarlane (*AF*), p. 209.

238 "*I learned yesterday . . .*": letter, October 7, 1944, J. F. Fulton to Dr. Per J. Hedenius, Yale, JFF 776.38.

239 "*became agitated . . .*": Abraham, *Chain.*

PROFOUNDLY DISTURBED . . . : cable, October 25, 1944, J. F. Fulton to Dr. Göran Liljestrand, Yale, JFF 776.40.

"*We are all much relieved . . .*": letter, November 8, 1944, J. F. Fulton to Dr. Göran Liljestrand, Yale, JFF 776.41.

240 Credit for oxygen: Carl Djerassi and Roald Hoffmann, *Oxygen* (Weinheim, Germany: Wiley-VCH, 2001). The play raises these questions and is an enlightening and entertaining examination of how credit is—and isn't—given.

241 "*It is clear . . .*": internal memo, April 8, 1943, Göran Liljestrand to other committee members, Nobel Archives.

NGH and Mercy Bing: Rose Heatley, "How We Met," 1994, Heatley family collection.

242 American production of penicillin: Helfand et al, "Wartime Industrial Production of Penicillin," p. 51.

"*A lot of literature . . .*": internal memo, July 20, 1944, Göran Liljestrand to other committee members, Nobel Archives.

"*indisputable . . . class as Fleming's*": internal memo, August 19, 1944, Nanna Svartz to Liljestrand, Nobel Archives.

242–43 Details of the Floreys' trip home: Charles Florey, interview with EL.

243 "*she found it hard . . .*": Paquita Florey McMichael, interview with EL.

"*There is a lot of axe grinding . . .*": letter, July 26, 1945, HWF to J. F. Fulton, Yale, JFF, 777.

244 "*I was more than ever . . .*": letter, August 4, 1945, J. F. Fulton to HWF, Yale, JFF 777/13.

"*You are a very good friend . . .*": letter, September 9, 1945, HWF to J. F. Fulton, Yale, JFF 777/15.

Paramount Pictures invitation: RS, 98 HF 36.15.

245 "*as we have . . .*": letter, July 2, 1945, HWF to Lord Moran, RS, 98 HF 36.15.4.

"*My 'good cause' . . .*": letter, July 5, 1945, Lord Moran to HWF, RS, 98 HF 36.15.5.

"I have had many compliments . . .": speech, Alexander Fleming, Fleming papers, British Library, 56123, vol. 17, lectures and speeches 1945–1946.
Fleming's appealing character: Macfarlane (*AF*), p. 260.
"My dear Liljestrand . . .": letter, January 8, 1945, Sir Henry Dale to Dr. Göran Liljestrand, RS, 93 HD 55.3.33.

246 Sven Hellerström: internal memo, August 31, 1945, Hellerström to Liljestrand, Nobel Archives.
"From this discovery . . .": internal memo, August 27, 1945, Anders Kristenson to Liljestrand, Nobel Archives.
"This year even more scientists . . .": internal memo, August 20, 1945, Göran Liljestrand to other Nobel committee members, Nobel Archives.

247 THE CAROLINE INSTITUTE . . . : telegram, Hilding Bergstrand to HWF, RS, 98 HF 289.16.9.
"Is it true . . .": *New York Times*, October 26, 1945.
NOBEL AWARD BRINGS . . . : cable, October 26, 1945, J. F. Fulton to Dr. Göran Liljestrand, Yale, JFF 777/17.
WARMEST CONGRATULATIONS . . . : cable, October 26, 1945, J. F. Fulton to Ernst Chain, Yale, JFF 777/24.

248 ALL IS WELL . . . : cable, October 26, 1945, J. F. Fulton to HWF, Yale, JFF 777/23.
CORRECTION IMPERATIVE . . . : telegram, October 26, 1945, J. F. Fulton to Editor, *New York Times*, Yale, JFF 777/21.

14: THE MAKERS OF GREAT MEDICINE

249 *"festivities . . . put a considerable . . ."*: letter, December 28, 1945, Ernst Chain to Perrin Long, Yale, JFF 777/32.
"I had the week of my life . . .": letter, December 17, 1945, Ethel Reed Florey to Lucia and John Fulton, Abraham, NCUACSs 103/2/02, D 71.

250 *"The Swedes really . . ."*: letter, December 28, 1945, HWF to J. F. Fulton and Lucia Fulton, Yale, JFF 777/31.

251 *"Fleming was the first . . ."*: W. Maxwell Cowan, interview with EL.
Chain's unhappiness with *Antibiotics*: Abraham, *Chain*.
Forum for Chain to argue: Clark, *Life of Chain*, p. 105.
British National Research Development Corporation: Macfarlane (*AF*), p. 206.
"It is often . . .": Sir Henry Harris, interview with EL.

252–53 *"My Dear Professor . . ."* and *". . . an episode . . ."*: Clark, *Life of Chain*, pp. 115–16.

253 *"I hope that your . . ."*: letter, September 26, 1949, HWF to Ernst Chain, RS, 98 HF 35.11.52.

254 Fleming's honors: Macfarlane (*AF*), pp. 289–92.
"ordinary people were sick . . .": Ibid., p. 260.

255 Feelings at Oxford about Fleming memorial and *"The ball has been passed . . ."*: RS, 98 HF 34.20.1–5.

256 *"I don't think . . .":* RS, 98 HF 34.20.4.

257 *"Each of them received . . .":* Ludovici, *Fleming, Discoverer of Penicillin,* p. 202.
     "Who is that codger . . .": Maxwell Cowan, interview with EL.
     "would rest . . ." and other details: Paquita Florey McMichael, interview with EL.
     "was not very relaxed . . .": Paquita Florey McMichael, interview with Dr. Max Blythe, Oxford Brookes University, the Royal College of Physicians and Oxford Brookes University Medical Sciences Video Archive.

258 *"Dad had a didactic . . .":* Paquita Florey McMichael, interview with EL.

259 *"Dear Mrs. Jennings . . .":* letter, November 3, 1966, HWF to Margaret Jennings, RS, 98 HF 297.10.17.

260 Abraham's offer of royalties: Mercy Heatley, interview with EL.

261 *"He said he likes . . .":* Ibid.
     "The committee recommends . . .": Henry Harris, interview with EL.

262 *"genome drugs are a long way . . ."* and number of new antibiotics, and details of antibiotics: Dr. John G. Bartlett, interview with EL.

BIBLIOGRAPHY

Baldry, Peter. *The Battle Against Bacteria: A Fresh Look*. Cambridge: Cambridge University Press, 1976.

Bickel, Lennard. *Rise Up to Life: A Biography of Howard Walter Florey Who Gave Penicillin to the World*. London: Angus and Robertson, 1972.

Brendon, Piers. *The Dark Valley: A Panorama of the 1930s*. New York: Alfred A. Knopf, 2000.

Bryson, Bill. *A Short History of Nearly Everything*. New York: Broadway Books, 2003.

Cantor, Norman F. *In the Wake of the Plague*. New York: The Free Press, 2001.

Carrell, Jennifer Lee. *The Speckled Monster: A Historical Tale of Battling Smallpox*. New York: Dutton, 2003.

Churchill, Winston. *Their Finest Hour*. New York: Houghton Mifflin Company, 1949.

Clark, Ronald W. *The Life of Ernst Chain: Penicillin and Beyond*. New York: St. Martin's Press, 1985.

Colebrook, Leonard. *Almroth Wright, Provocative Doctor and Thinker*. London: William Heinemann, 1954.

Djerassi, Carl, and Roald Hoffmann. *Oxygen*. Weinheim, Germany: Wiley-VCH, 2001.

Dowling, Harry F. *Fighting Infection, Conquests of the Twentieth Century*. Cambridge: Harvard University Press, 1977, 2000.

Dunnill, Michael. *The Plato of Praed Street: The Life and Times of Almroth Wright*. London: The Royal Society of Medicine Press, 2002.

Florey, H. W., E. Chain, N. G. Heatley, M. A. Jennings, A. G. Sanders, E. P. Abraham, and M. E. Florey. *Antibiotics* (2 volumes). London: Oxford University Press, 1949.

Gardner, A. D. *Some Recollections*. Bound typescript in the University College Library, Oxford University, 1975.

Garfield, Simon. *Mauve*. London: Faber and Faber, 2000.

Hare, Ronald. *The Birth of Penicillin*. London: George Allen and Unwin, 1970.

Harris, Henry. *The Balance of Improbabilities.* Oxford: Oxford University Press, 1987.

Helfand, W. H., H. B. Woodruff, K. M. H. Coleman et al. "Wartime Industrial Development of Penicillin in the United States." In *The History of Antibiotics: A Symposium,* ed. John Parascandola. Madison: American Institute of the History of Pharmacy, 1980.

Hobby, Gladys L. *Penicillin: Meeting the Challenge.* New Haven: Yale University Press, 1985.

Hoffmann, Roald. *The Same and Not the Same.* New York: Columbia University Press, 1995.

Hoffmann, Roald, and Vivian Torrence. *Chemistry Imagined: Reflections on Science.* Washington, D.C. and London: Smithsonian Institution Press, 1993.

Hughes, W. Howard. *Alexander Fleming and Penicillin.* Hove, Sussex: Priory Press, 1974.

Isaacson, Walter. *Benjamin Franklin: An American Life.* New York: Simon and Schuster, 2003.

Jenkins, Roy. *Winston Churchill, A Biography.* New York: Farrar, Straus and Giroux, 2001.

Jonas, Gerald. *The Circuit Riders: Rockefeller Money and the Rise of Modern Science.* New York: W. W. Norton and Company, 1989.

Keegan, John. *Winston Churchill.* New York: Viking, 2002.

Ludovici, L. J. *Fleming, Discoverer of Penicillin.* London: Andrew Dakers, Science Book Club Edition, 1952.

Macfarlane, Gwyn. *Alexander Fleming: The Man and the Myth.* Cambridge: Harvard University Press, 1984.

———. *Howard Florey: The Making of a Great Scientist.* Oxford: Oxford University Press, 1979.

Mann, John. *The Elusive Magic Bullet: The Search for the Perfect Drug.* Oxford: Oxford University Press, 1999.

Masters, David. *Miracle Drug.* London: Eyre and Spottiswoode, 1946.

Maurois, André. *The Life of Sir Alexander Fleming, Discoverer of Penicillin.* Trans. Gerard Hopkins. New York: E. P. Dutton and Company, 1959.

McNeill, William H. *Plagues and Peoples.* New York: Anchor Books, 1998.

Moberg, Carol L., and Zanvil A. Cohn, eds. *Launching the Antibiotic Era.* New York: The Rockefeller University Press, 1990.

Porter, Roy. *The Greatest Benefit to Mankind.* New York: W. W. Norton and Company, 1998.

Ratcliff, J. D. *Yellow Magic.* New York: Random House, 1945.

Riordan, Michael, and Lillian Hoddeston. *Crystal Fire: The Invention of the Transistor and the Birth of the Information Age.* Sloan Technology Series. New York: W. W. Norton and Company, 1997.

Root-Bernstein, Robert Scott. *Discovering.* Cambridge: Harvard University Press, 1989.

Williams, Trevor I. *Howard Florey: Penicillin and After.* London: Oxford University Press, 1984.

———. *Robert Robinson, Chemist Extraordinary.* Oxford: Oxford University Press, 1990.

———. *Science: A History of Discovery in the Twentieth Century.* Oxford: Oxford University Press, 1990.

Wilson, David. *In Search of Penicillin.* New York: Alfred A. Knopf, 1976.

RESEARCH

Yale University: Manuscripts and Archives, Sterling Memorial Library, and Historical Library, Cushing/Whitney Medical Library, New Haven, Connecticut.

Nobel Archives, Karolinska Institutet, Stockholm, Sweden.

Bodleian Library, Oxford University, Oxford, England.

National Library of Australia, Canberra.

Wellcome Library for the History and Understanding of Medicine, the Wellcome Trust, London.

The British Library, London.

UCLA Medical Library, Los Angeles, California.

Oxford Brookes University, the Royal College of Physicians and Oxford Brookes University Medical Sciences Video Archives, Oxford, England.

The House of Lords Records Office (The Parliamentary Archives), London.

The Rockefeller Foundation Archives, the Rockefeller Archive Center, Sleepy Hollow, New York.

Pfizer Archives, Sandwich, Kent, England.

National Catalogue Unit for Archives of Contemporary Scientists, University of Bath, Bath, England.

The Royal Society Library, London.

ACKNOWLEDGMENTS

I read obituaries. They are a way to say good-bye to someone known or to meet someone new, if only at the last moment. Anne Miller was one of the new. After I finished Wolfgang Saxon's account of her life in the *New York Times* in June 1999, I wondered: Why did it take twelve years from Alexander Fleming's notice of penicillin's effect to the production of a drug that changed the course of human health, and why did Howard Florey and his group develop it and not Fleming? A few days later, I was having dinner in London with Colin Webb, who has published two of my books in England. Colin had heard of Mrs. Miller's obituary and the curious course of penicillin via Alistair Cooke's weekly *Letter from America* broadcast on the BBC; it would make an interesting book, he said. I thank him for a boost at just the right moment.

I am grateful that my agent Owen Laster and Jack Macrae of Holt were as intrigued as I. Owen's persistence and Jack's enthusiasm made for a happy partnership. My thanks as well to Jonathan Pecarsky at William Morris and to Katy Hope, Supurna Banerjee, and Christopher O'Connell at Holt. Thanks also to Alan Sampson and Little, Brown in London for their early support and to Ursula Mackenzie and Stephen Guise for their later help.

Libraries and archives provide the foundation and infrastructure for a book like this, and I am indebted to the British Library; the Bodleian Library, Oxford University; the Wellcome Library for the History and Understanding of Medicine, the Wellcome Trust, London; the Medical Library of the University of California, Los Angeles; Andrew Pitt and the Pfizer Archives, Sandwich, Kent; Jennie Lynch and the House of Lords Records Office (The Parliamentary Archives), London; Christine Ritchie and the University College Library, Oxford University; Kevin Brown and the St. Mary's Hospital Archives, London; Dr. Carol Beadle and Oxford Brookes University, the Royal College of Physicians and Oxford Brookes University Medical Sciences Video Archive, Oxford; Natasha Hennoste and the National Library of Australia, Canberra; Nancy F. Lyon and Manuscripts and Archives, Sterling Memorial Library, and Toby Appel, Ph.D., MLS, Historical Library, Cushing/Whitney Medical Library, Yale University, New Haven, Connecticut; Ann-Margareth Jörnvall and the Nobel Archives, Stockholm; Dr. Erwin Levold and the Rockefeller Foundation Archives, the Rockefeller Archive Center, Sleepy Hollow, New York; and Dr. Peter Harper, Dr. Tim Powell, Caroline Thibeaud, and the National Catalogue Unit for Archives of Contemporary Scientists, University of Bath, Somerset, England. Material from the Nobel Archives was kindly provided by the Nobel Committee for Physiology or Medicine. For translations, my thanks to Ann-Sofie Johansson.

I spent several months in the glorious library of the Royal Society. The cherubs that flit about in the fresco on the ceiling of the main reading room—which looks out through tall windows into St. James's Park—are a clue that this is Archive Heaven. Not that a clue is needed. I was made welcome and helped at every turn by Clara Anderson, Rupert Baker, Martin Carr, Joanna Corden, Gillian Jackson, Stephanie Morris, Karen Peters, Gudrun Richardson, Heather Smithson, and Christine Wollett. They have my unending thanks and appreciation. Thanks as well to Teresa Bezzina for always keeping the door open.

For help in tracking down and collecting information in England, I thank Pam Kent, who introduced me to Laura Chapman, who passed me on to Brigid Buckman, who put me in the hands of the wonderfully capable Emma Farrer Bravo. Thanks as well to Dr. Michael T. Bravo of Downing College, Cambridge, for a helpful reading of several chapters and for enlisting the aid of Dr. Brian Dolan and Professor Dorothy Porter of the Department of Anthropology, History, and Social Medicine, University of California, San Francisco. I appreciate their suggestions. For their time and recollections I thank Sir Aaron Klug, Dr. Benjamin Chain, Dr. John G. Bartlett, Dr. Robert Scott Root-Bernstein, Megan Lancaster Nurser and John Nurser, and Ruth Callow Parker and Bob Parker.

Friends in London—Marion Underhill, Warren and Olivia Hoge, Rachel Billington, Ben Hooberman, and Jane Spender—made being away almost like being at home. Doug Hayward, the Tailor of Mount Street, and Audie Charles provided a package drop, tea, and easy conversation. Thanks as well to Gina Glennon, Lee Madden, and all at J. Sheekey for a ready table.

I am grateful to Professor Sir Henry Harris, who succeeded Howard Florey as Professor of Pathology at Oxford. His personal acquaintance with the principals of the story gave me an invaluable, authoritative insight into the character and contribution of each. Thanks also to Colin Ryde, Dr. Siamon Gordon, Dr. George Brownlee, and Pam Woodward of the Sir William Dunn School of Pathology. My fond thanks to Gina Pattison and Nick Beloff for their help and wonderful company in both Oxford and London.

Charles and Sue Florey and Paquita Florey McMichael graciously opened their homes and their memories to me and allowed me unfettered access to family papers. My warmest thanks for their inestimable help and kindness.

Norman Heatley spent many hours over many months recounting the details of his work and that of others on the Oxford team. He was a pleasurable companion and a generous one as well. His personal diaries, unavailable for research until now, are a time machine that brings immediacy to the story that it otherwise could not have. My admiration for him is unbounded. The world has lost a lovely man. Mercy Heatley suggested avenues of research, introduced me to key people, and fed me well besides.

She has my fondest thanks. Their daughter Rose Heatley gave me family papers and a sense of her parents, and I thank her for her thoughtful help.

As do all who knew him, I mourn the death of W. Maxwell Cowan. His early encouragement was a boon. I am grateful to Kenneth Turan for pointing me toward the title, and to the Honorable Andreas Eckman and the Honorable Anita Eckman for ushering me into the Nobel Archives.

My gratitude to Mona Golabeck, the spectacularly talented pianist, radio host, and author of *The Children of Willesden Lane*, the story of her mother's rescue by the Kindertransport. She is also my friend. Her winning bid for this space provided a generous contribution to PEN Center USA West.

Affectionate thanks to David Wolf for many readings of chapters and for enduring my whining when the writing was slow. For reading the manuscript and for constant kindnesses, the same thanks to my friends William Tyrer (who always worried about the page count), Walter Hill, Linda Tyrer, Edward Dolnick, Linda "Sherlock" Amster, Peter Tauber, Jim Trickett, April Smith, Larry Chernikoff, Anne Wadsworth, and my brother-in-law, the amazing polymath Joseph G. Perpich. In separate acts of great friendship, K. C. Cole introduced me to *Oxygen* and helped to let the air in, and Jonathan Segal knew just what to do.

Arthur Ochs Sulzberger and Allison Cowles let me use their London flat so often that the neighbors thought I was a tenant. My abiding love and thanks to them.

My wife, Karen Sulzberger, and our sons, Simon and John, gamely put up with absences I hated to take (especially during vacations), however beguiling my research or imminent the deadline. Their love is a constant buoy, and mine for them is in every word.

INDEX

ABOUT THE AUTHOR

Eric Lax's books include the international bestseller *Woody Allen, A Biography*, and the award-winning *Life and Death on 10 West*, an account of the patients, doctors, and nurses on the UCLA bone marrow transplantation ward; both were *New York Times* Notable Books. His work has appeared in many magazines and newspapers, including *The New York Times Magazine, Vanity Fair, The Atlantic, Life*, and *Esquire*. He lives in Los Angeles with his wife and two sons.